Tassilo Marchetti

Hormone therapies

Science, application and perspectives

bup

Tassilo Marchetti

Hormone therapies

Science, application and perspectives

Print: ISBN 978-3-69035-248-2
eBook: ISBN: 978-3-69035-256-7

Order number: 1847
Also available as an eBook

Bremen University Press
Fahrenheitstr. 11
D-28359 Bremen

bup@bremenuniversitypress.com
www.bremenuniversitypress.com

Tassilo Marchetti

Hormone therapies

Science, application and perspectives

Overview

Table of contents

Introduction

Clarification of terms

Hormone therapy is a medical treatment in which hormones are administered or regulated to influence physiological processes, treat diseases or alleviate symptoms. Hormones are chemical messengers that are produced by endocrine glands and control a variety of biological functions in the body, including metabolism , growth , reproduction and mood regulation. Depending on the objective, hormone therapy can take different forms and be used in different areas.

Hormone therapy is basically divided into two main categories: the administration of hormones and the blocking or regulation of the body's own hormone production.

The former is often used when there is a hormonal imbalance or a hormone deficiency , such as in substitution therapy. Typical examples of this are the administration of insulin for diabetes mellitus, the administration of thyroid hormones for an underactive thyroid (hypothyroidism) or hormone replacement therapy (hormone replacement therapy) for post-menopausal women to alleviate menopausal symptoms.

The second variant, in which the effect of hormones is blocked or modulated, is particularly relevant in oncology , especially for hormone-dependent tumours such as breast or prostate cancer . This involves the use of substances that either inhibit the production of certain hormones or block their effect on the target cells. Such treatments can slow down or stop the growth of hormone-dependent tumour cells.

Hormone therapy is also used in other medical contexts. In reproductive medicine , it is used to regulate the menstrual cycle , promote egg maturation or trigger ovulation . In transgender medicine it supports the process of gender reassignment, for example by administering testosterone or oestrogens to adapt the secondary sexual characteristics to the desired gender.

Despite its wide range of uses, hormone therapy is not free of risks and side effects . Treatment requires careful consideration of the risk-benefit balance and continuous monitoring. Possible side effects include thrombosis, metabolic disorders, an increased tendency to develop cancer in certain contexts and adverse effects on the cardiovascular system. The choice of suitable hormones, dosages and forms of administration is therefore crucial for the success and safety of the therapy.

Hormone therapy is a versatile and effective medical treatment strategy that is used specifically in a variety of clinical pictures. Its application is based on a sound understanding of endocrine regulation and requires individualised adaptation to the needs and health conditions of the patient.

Historical overview

The history of hormone therapy is closely linked to the discovery and understanding of hormones, which are chemical messengers that control numerous physiological processes in the body. The first indications of hormonal mechanisms of action date back to the 19th century, when Arnold Berthold demonstrated through experiments with castrated cockerels that glands secrete substances that influence the development of organisms. The term "hormone" was coined in 1905 by Ernest Starling and William Bayliss, who described the chemical transmission of signals between organs. The therapeutic effect of glandular extracts was recognised early on, for example in the treatment of hypothyroidism or the first successful use of insulin to treat diabetes in 1921. The discovery and isolation of hormones such as cortisone, oestrogen , progesterone and testosterone in the 1930s led to the development of specific hormonal therapies. This revolutionised the treatment of numerous diseases such as rheumatoid arthritis, hormone-dependent cancers and menopausal symptoms. The development of oral contraceptives in the 1950s marked a social and medical milestone by giving women control over their reproduction. With the advancement of biotechnology in the 1980s, synthetically produced hormones became available that offered greater purity and efficacy. In modern medicine, hormone therapy can be used in a variety of ways, for example in oncology , reproductive medicine or gender medicine. Newer approaches rely on personalised therapies, bioidentical hormones and the use of recombinant technologies to increase the precision and safety of treatment. This continuous development shows the central role of hormone therapy in medicine and its potential for future innovations.

Relevance of the topic

Hormone therapies are of central importance from a medical, social and scientific perspective, as they regulate a wide range of functions in the human body and can treat numerous diseases or alleviate symptoms. From a medical perspective, they enable the targeted correction of hormonal imbalances caused by endocrine disorders, natural ageing processes or diseases. They are essential for the treatment of chronic diseases such as diabetes mellitus, hypothyroidism or osteoporosis , but also for the treatment of hormone-dependent tumours such as breast and prostate cancer . They also play an important role in reproductive medicine and offer people with an unfulfilled desire to have children effective options. Socially, hormone therapies contribute to improving the quality of life, particularly for women during and after the menopause , for transgender people in the context of gender reassignment and through the development of hormonal contraceptives , which have revolutionised family planning. However, their importance goes beyond individual benefits, as they have also triggered social discussions about gender, reproduction and health. From a scientific perspective, hormone therapies promote research into complex endocrine networks and drive innovation in biotechnology, for example through the development of synthetic or recombinant hormones. These advances not only contribute to better treatment options, but also open up new perspectives in personalised medicine by allowing therapies to be tailored more precisely to the genetic and molecular characteristics of the individual. Overall, hormone therapies are an indispensable part of modern medicine, as they promote individual health as well as advancing social and scientific developments.

Part I: Basics of hormone therapy

Biochemistry and physiology of hormones

Hormones are chemical messengers that are produced by specialised cells, usually in endocrine glands, and released into the bloodstream to influence distant target cells. They regulate numerous physiological processes such as growth, metabolism, reproduction and homeostasis. Biochemically, hormones can be categorised into three main classes: Peptide hormones, steroid hormones and amino acid derivatives. Peptide hormones, such as insulin and glucagon, consist of amino acid chains, while steroid hormones such as cortisol and oestrogen are derived from cholesterol. Amino acid derivatives, such as adrenaline and thyroxine, are created by modifying individual amino acids.

Hormones are produced in specialised endocrine glands, such as the pituitary gland, thyroid gland, adrenal glands or the sex glands. These glands are regulated by a complex network of feedback mechanisms that enable precise control of hormone levels. The hypothalamus plays a central role in this by influencing the pituitary gland and subsequently peripheral endocrine glands via releasing or inhibiting hormones. For example, the release of thyroid hormones is controlled by the hypothalamic-pituitary-thyroid axis.

Hormones act via specific receptors on or in target cells. These receptors are highly specific for certain hormones and can be localised either on the membrane or intracellularly. Water-soluble hormones such as peptide hormones bind to receptors on the cell surface as they cannot pass through the cell membrane. This receptor binding activates signal transduction pathways, usually via G-protein -coupled receptors or tyrosine kinases , which mobilise secondary messengers such as cAMP or calcium and thus trigger a cascade of intracellular reactions. Lipophilic hormones such as steroid hormones and thyroid hormones , on the other hand, can diffuse through the cell membrane and bind to intracellular receptors. The hormone-receptor complex enters the cell nucleus, where it directly influences gene expression and thus triggers long-term effects such as protein biosynthesis .

The hormone effect is regulated at several levels: In addition to the synthesis and secretion of hormones, transport proteins , receptor density and the activation or inhibition of downstream signalling pathways also play a role. Homeostasis is ensured via negative feedback loops, such as the inhibition of hypothalamic hormones by peripheral hormone levels . Positive feedback is less common, but occurs, for example, during ovulation or during labour.

To summarise, hormones are essential regulators of the body whose function is based on precise biochemistry, complex physiological regulation and specific signal transduction mechanisms. This interplay enables adaptation to changing internal and external conditions and forms the basis for hormonal control of the body's diverse functions.

Diagnosis of hormonal disorders

The diagnosis of hormonal disorders is an essential part of endocrinological medicine today, as hormonal imbalances can cause a variety of symptoms and diseases. Diagnostics includes biochemical measurements, imaging procedures and genetic analyses in order to identify the underlying causes and determine the optimal therapy.

Methods of hormone measurement

The central method for diagnosing hormonal disorders is the determination of hormone levels in various body fluids.

Blood tests

Blood tests are the most frequently used method for diagnosing hormonal disorders, as they enable accurate and reliable quantification of hormone concentrations. They offer a wide range of applications to assess basal hormone levels as well as their regulation and responsiveness to external stimuli. Thyroid hormones such as triiodothyronine (T3), thyroxine (T4) and thyroid stimulating hormone (TSH) are routinely measured to assess thyroid function . Elevated or decreased levels of these hormones provide information about diseases such as hypothyroidism or hyperthyroidism and their possible causes, such as autoimmune diseases or iodine deficiency . Sex hormones such as oestrogen , testosterone and progesterone are also frequently analysed, particularly in cases of infertility , cycle disorders, puberty problems or hormone therapies. Their levels enable a differentiated diagnosis of disorders of gonadal function, hormonal imbalances during the menopause or hypogonadism .

The measurement of adrenal hormones such as cortisol and aldosterone is central to the diagnosis of diseases such as Cushing's syndrome , adrenal insufficiency or Conn's syndrome . Cortisol levels can be checked as part of a dexamethasone inhibition test or an ACTH stimulation test to assess the function of the hypothalamic-pituitary-adrenal axis. Aldosterone is often measured in combination with renin to assess the renin-angiotensin-aldosterone system, especially in cases of hypertension or electrolyte disturbances .

Pancreatic hormones such as insulin and glucagon are also taken into account in hormone analysis. Insulin levels are essential for the diagnosis and monitoring of diabetes mellitus or insulin resistance , while glucagon is relevant in the assessment of hypoglycaemic conditions or pancreatic tumours. Blood tests enable not only the measurement of absolute hormone levels , but also the investigation of dynamic processes by recording the reaction of the endocrine system to specific stimuli or inhibitions. Stimulation tests , such as the ACTH stimulation test or the glucose tolerance test , and suppression tests, such as the dexamethasone inhibition test, provide decisive indications of dysfunctions within complex hormonal control circuits. These procedures provide a precise basis for diagnosis and the planning of individualised therapies.

Saliva tests

Saliva tests play an increasingly important role in the monitoring and adjustment of hormone therapies as they provide a precise and non-invasive method to determine free, biologically active hormone levels . In contrast to serum tests , where a large proportion of the hormones are bound to transport proteins and therefore do not directly reflect the bioactive fraction, analysing saliva allows direct measurement of those hormones that are actually active at target tissues. This makes it particularly valuable for the fine-tuning of hormone therapies.

A key area of application for saliva tests is in the treatment of sex hormones such as oestrogen , progesterone and testosterone , for example in menopausal women or in men with testosterone deficiency. The measurement of salivary hormones makes it possible to monitor the effects of the administered hormones on the bioavailable levels in the body. This means that overdoses can be avoided and side effects minimised. It also ensures that the dosage is sufficient to achieve therapeutic effects without unnecessarily burdening the hormone balance.

Saliva analysis has also proven to be useful when treating with adrenal hormones , such as cortisol or DHEA. It is particularly important to regularly monitor the effect of substituted hormones in patients with adrenal insufficiency or chronic stress. Saliva tests offer the possibility of mapping circadian fluctuations and thus developing an individualised dosing strategy that is based on the natural hormonal rhythms . This precise adjustment is crucial to prevent both an undersupply and an overdose, which could lead to significant health problems in the long term.

Another advantage of saliva tests for hormone therapies is the possibility of self-administration. Patients can take samples conveniently at home, which significantly increases acceptance and compliance. This is particularly important for long-term therapies where regular checks are required. The ease of use and the ability to take samples at different times of the day allow comprehensive and detailed monitoring, which would be difficult to realise in clinical settings with blood samples.

Saliva tests also contribute to the optimisation of personalised medicine, as they enable doctors to tailor treatment to the individual needs of the patient. This is particularly relevant in the case of complex hormonal disorders, where standard doses are often insufficient or can cause undesirable effects. By regularly monitoring the free hormone levels in saliva, treatment plans can be

dynamically adapted to achieve the best possible therapeutic success.

Urine analyses

The 24-hour urine collection test is an established
method for assessing hormone excretion and provides
valuable diagnostic information, particularly for steroid
hormones such as cortisol or catecholamines . In contrast
to selective measurements in blood or saliva, this
method allows an integrative recording of hormonal activity over a longer period of time. As a result, fluctuations in hormone levels caused by the circadian rhythm
or acute stress reactions can be compensated for, enabling a more comprehensive assessment of hormonal
status.

The 24-hour urine collection test plays a central role in
the analysis of steroid hormones such as cortisol , particularly in the diagnosis of diseases such as Cushing's syndrome or adrenal insufficiency . By measuring the total
amount of free cortisol excreted in the urine throughout
the day, indications of hyper- or hypofunction of the adrenal glands can be obtained. This method is particularly
useful for identifying subtle disorders that might be
missed by a single blood or saliva sample.

The 24-hour urine collection sample is also a crucial diagnostic tool when analysing catecholamines such as
adrenaline , noradrenaline and their metabolites, for example vanillin mandelic acid . These hormones, which

play an important role in the stress response and the regulation of the cardiovascular system, are released episodically, which makes the interpretation of individual measurements difficult. The 24-hour collection makes it possible to average these fluctuations and obtain a more accurate picture of catecholaminergic activity. This is particularly important in the diagnosis of tumours such as pheochromocytomas , which cause excessive production of these hormones.

The 24-hour urine collection sample also has advantages in the evaluation of the effect and monitoring of hormone therapies. It offers an opportunity to monitor the effect of administered hormones or their precursors over a longer period of time. Particularly in patients who are being treated with steroid hormones or catecholamine-like substances, this method can help to optimise the therapy and avoid undesirable side effects due to over- or underdosing.

Although the method is considered reliable and informative, it is not without its challenges. The correct collection of urine over 24 hours requires a high level of patient compliance. Incorrect sampling or incomplete collections can falsify the results. Nevertheless, this method remains an important diagnostic tool, particularly in endocrinology, as it provides a comprehensive insight into the body's hormonal activity.

Imaging

Imaging techniques such as ultrasound , computed tomography (CT), magnetic resonance imaging (MRI) and scintigraphy are key diagnostic tools for detecting structural abnormalities in hormone-producing organs. These methods complement biochemical analyses and enable precise localisation and characterisation of changes that can cause hormonal imbalances, such as tumours or other pathological processes.

Ultrasound is often used as a first-line test, particularly when examining the thyroid gland . It offers a non-invasive and radiation-free way of assessing the size, structure and any nodules of the thyroid gland. With modern high-resolution devices, even small lesions can be detected and assessed for their echogenic properties, which can indicate whether they are benign or malignant. In addition, Doppler sonography can be used to analyse the blood flow in thyroid nodules or other suspicious tissue.

Computed tomography (CT) plays an important role in the assessment of hormone-producing organs such as the adrenal glands . It provides detailed cross-sectional images that are helpful in identifying tumours, cysts or other changes. CT is particularly useful in the evaluation of adrenal adenomas or carcinomas as it can accurately depict the size, density and morphological characteristics of lesions. It is also frequently used in the staging diagnosis of tumours to identify possible metastases.

Magnetic resonance imaging (MRI) is another highly specialised procedure that has proven particularly useful for examining the pituitary gland . As the pituitary gland is a small but extremely important hormone-producing organ in the skull, MRI, with its excellent soft tissue imaging, offers the possibility of visualising microadenomas or other structural anomalies associated with hormonal dysfunctions such as acromegaly, Cushing's disease or prolactin omene. Compared to CT, MRI has the advantage that it does not require ionising radiation, which makes it suitable for repeated examinations.

Scintigraphy is a functional imaging procedure that is primarily used in endocrinology. In the thyroid gland it is used to identify so-called "hot" or "cold" nodules, which is crucial for differentiating between benign and potentially malignant lesions. In adrenal gland diagnostics, scintigraphy can be used to localise functional tumours such as pheochromocytomas or hormone-active adenomas . It offers the advantage of evaluating not only the structure but also the function of the organs, which is particularly important when planning a therapy.

These imaging procedures are indispensable components in the diagnosis of diseases of hormone-producing organs. They provide detailed information about the anatomy and function of these organs and thus enable a precise diagnosis to be made. By using them, structural anomalies such as tumours, cysts or hyperplasia can be effectively detected and the basis for further therapeutic decisions can be created.

Typical symptoms and their interpretation

Hormonal disorders often manifest themselves in non-specific symptoms that require careful clinical evaluation. Examples of typical symptoms and their hormonal causes are as follows.

Exhaustion and weight gain

Fatigue and weight gain are often non-specific symptoms, but they can indicate serious endocrine disorders such as hypothyroidism or adrenal insufficiency . Both disorders are characterised by impaired hormonal regulation, which can have a significant impact on the entire metabolism , energy production and general well-being.

Hypothyroidism , an underactive thyroid gland , is one of the most common causes of this combination of symptoms. It is caused by reduced production of the thyroid hormones T3 (triiodothyronine) and T4 (thyroxine), which play a central role in the regulation of energy metabolism, heat production and the function of almost all organ systems. A deficiency of these hormones leads to a slowdown in metabolism, which can manifest itself in the form of weight gain , even with unchanged or reduced calorie consumption. Exhaustion occurs because the body has less energy available, which impairs both physical and mental activities. Other accompanying symptoms may include sensitivity to cold , dry skin , hair loss , constipation and depressive moods . Laboratory diagnosis is confirmed by determining the thyroid-stimulating hormone (TSH) and the free thyroid hormones fT3 and fT4. An elevated TSH value with simultaneously reduced fT3 and/or fT4 indicates primary hypothyroidism, while a central cause, such as a pituitary disorder, can be suspected by other specific constellations.

Adrenal insufficiency , which can be either primary (Addison's disease) or secondary (pituitary-related), is another possible cause of fatigue and weight gain . In this disease, the production of cortisol , an important stress hormone of the adrenal cortex, is insufficient. Cortisol is significantly involved in the regulation of metabolic processes, the immune response and coping with stress. A deficiency leads to general physical weakness and chronic fatigue, as the body is unable to react appropriately to physical or psychological stress. Weight gain is often a consequence of secondary processes, such as increased water retention due to accompanying electrolyte disorders or a reduced mobilisation of fatty acids and glucose from energy stores. In addition, symptoms such as low blood pressure, salt cravings, hyperpigmentation of the skin and gastrointestinal complaints may occur. The diagnosis is confirmed by measuring the morning serum cortisol and, if necessary, by an ACTH stimulation test. A low cortisol level in combination with an elevated ACTH level indicates primary adrenal insufficiency, while a normal or low ACTH level suggests a secondary cause.

A laboratory diagnosis is essential here in order to identify the underlying cause of the symptoms and initiate targeted therapy. While hypothyroidism is usually treated with thyroid hormone substitution such as levothyroxine , adrenal insufficiency requires the administration of glucocorticoids and, in some cases, mineralocorticoids. Early diagnosis and treatment are crucial to alleviate symptoms and avoid long-term complications.

Unintentional weight loss , nervousness and palpitations

Unwanted weight loss , nervousness and palpitations are classic symptoms of hyperthyroidism , an overactive thyroid gland , in which there is excessive production of the thyroid hormones triiodothyronine (T3) and thyroxine (T4). These hormones play a central role in the regulation of metabolism, heart function and nervous system activity. An excess leads to an acceleration of these processes, which manifests itself in the symptoms mentioned.

Unintentional weight loss occurs even though food intake is often unchanged or even increased. This is due to the increased metabolic activity, which leads to increased energy consumption. The body burns fat reserves and often also muscle mass to cover the increased energy requirement. In addition, thermogenesis is increased, which contributes to increased heat production and further calorie burning.

The nervousness and inner restlessness are the result of overstimulation of the sympathetic nervous system by the thyroid hormones . Those affected often report increased irritability, sleep disorders and a general inability to relax. These symptoms can have a significant impact on quality of life and are often the reason why patients seek medical advice.

Heart palpitations, medically known as tachycardia, are caused by the direct effect of the thyroid hormones on the cardiovascular system. They increase the heart rate, increase the contractility of the heart muscle and can lead to cardiac arrhythmias such as atrial fibrillation. These effects increase the heart's oxygen and energy requirements and can lead to heart failure in the long term if the hyperthyroidism is not treated.

The laboratory diagnosis is confirmed by measuring the thyroid hormones T3 and T4 as well as thyroid stimulating hormone (TSH). Hyperthyroidism is characterised by elevated levels of T3 and T4 in combination with a suppressed TSH value. This is an expression of negative feedback: the high hormone levels suppress the release of TSH by the pituitary gland . To further clarify the cause, the determination of thyroid autoantibodies, such as TRAK (TSH receptor antibodies), can be helpful. These are often elevated in Graves' disease , the most common cause of hyperthyroidism. In the case of thyroid nodules or autonomous adenomas , a scintigraphy of the thyroid gland can provide additional information.

The treatment of hyperthyroidism depends on the underlying cause. Options include medication to inhibit thyroid hormone synthesis using thyreostatic drugs such as thiamazole or propylthiouracil , radioiodine therapy or surgical removal of the thyroid gland . Symptomatic measures such as the administration of beta-blockers can help to control the heart rate and alleviate nervous symptoms. Early diagnosis and treatment are crucial to alleviate symptoms and avoid serious complications such as a thyrotoxic crisis.

Menstrual disorders and infertility

Menstrual irregularities and infertility are common problems that are often caused by a dysregulation of the sex hormones. These hormones, in particular oestrogen , progesterone , luteinising hormone (LH) and follicle stimulating hormone (FSH), are essential for the female cycle and reproductive capacity. A disruption in the hormonal balance can significantly impair the normal function of the ovaries and the regulation of the menstrual cycle .

Dysregulation of the sex hormones can manifest itself in various ways. A lack of oestrogen and progesterone can lead to irregular or absent menstrual bleeding. An overproduction of oestrogen, often accompanied by a lack of progesterone , on the other hand, can lead to excessively heavy or prolonged bleeding. Disorders in the secretion of LH and FSH , which are released from the pituitary gland , can prevent or delay ovulation , which severely restricts fertility.

A common syndrome associated with menstrual irregularities and infertility is polycystic ovary syndrome (PCOS). PCOS is a complex endocrine disorder characterised by an overproduction of androgens (male hormones), insulin resistance and impaired follicle maturation in the ovaries. Typical symptoms include irregular or absent menstrual cycles, anovulatory cycles (lack of ovulation), weight gain , acne and increased body hair growth (hirsutism). Ovarian dysfunction leads to an accumulation of immature follicles in the ovaries, which are visible on ultrasound as so-called "cysts ".

The diagnosis of menstrual disorders and infertility begins with a detailed medical history and a physical examination, followed by a laboratory diagnostic analysis of the relevant hormone levels. This includes the determination of oestrogen , progesterone , LH, FSH , prolactin and androgens such as testosterone as well as the thyroid hormones TSH and fT4, as thyroid dysfunction can also cause similar symptoms. An elevated LH/FSH quotient may indicate PCOS , while elevated prolactin levels may indicate hyperprolactinaemia as the cause of cycle disorders. Insulin resistance , which is often present in PCOS, is detected by measuring fasting insulin and glucose levels or by an oral glucose tolerance test .

In addition to laboratory diagnostics, diagnostic imaging, in particular transvaginal sonography, provides important information. It can assess the structure of the ovaries and identify typical features of PCOS , such as enlarged ovaries with multiple small cysts . If other structural abnormalities such as uterine fibroids or endometriosis are suspected, advanced diagnostic imaging or diagnostic laparoscopy may be necessary.

Treatment depends on the underlying cause and the individual needs of the patient. For PCOS , lifestyle changes such as weight reduction and regular physical activity are the main focus, as they can improve insulin resistance and hormonal status. Medication options include the administration of metformin to improve insulin resistance and the use of ovulation inducers such as clomiphene or letrozole to promote ovulation . For women who are not trying to conceive, hormonal contraception with combined oral contraceptives can help to regulate the cycle and alleviate symptoms of hyperandrogenism.

In cases caused by other hormonal dysregulations, specific therapy is required, such as hormone replacement for hypogonadism or drug inhibition of prolactin secretion for hyperprolactinaemia. Careful diagnosis and customised therapy are crucial to alleviate symptoms and restore fertility, if desired.

Bone fractures and muscle weakness

Bone fractures and muscle weakness can indicate hormonal disorders that affect bone metabolism and muscle strength. The most common causes include hormonal osteoporosis due to oestrogen deficiency, particularly during the menopause , and hyperparathyroidism , which is characterised by excessive production of parathyroid hormone (PTH).

Hormonal osteoporosis often develops as a result of oestrogen deficiency, as occurs during the menopause . Oestrogen plays a central role in bone metabolism as it inhibits the breakdown of bone tissue by osteoclasts and promotes the formation of new bone by osteoblasts . A lack of oestrogen leads to an imbalance between bone resorption and bone formation, with resorption being predominant. The resulting decrease in bone density increases the risk of fractures, particularly in the spine, hips and wrists. Clinically, this often manifests itself in the form of spontaneous or minor traumatic fractures. Muscle weakness often accompanies this, as the oestrogen deficiency can also have a negative impact on muscle metabolism, which further increases the risk of falling and therefore the risk of fractures .

Hyperparathyroidism , an overactive parathyroid gland, is another significant cause of bone fractures and muscle weakness . This disease leads to excessive secretion of parathyroid hormone , which regulates calcium levels in the blood. Chronically elevated PTH levels promote the breakdown of bone tissue to release calcium from the bones into the blood. This leads to a reduction in bone density and a weakening of the bone structure, which favours fractures. In addition, the disturbed calcium metabolism can lead to muscle weakness, as calcium is essential for muscle contraction. Patients with hyperparathyroidism often complain of generalised muscle weakness, fatigue and diffuse bone pain.

The diagnosis of these conditions requires careful laboratory diagnostics and imaging. If hormonal osteoporosis is suspected , bone density is measured using dual X-ray absorptiometry (DXA). In addition, serum levels of calcium, vitamin D and parathyroid hormone should be checked to rule out secondary osteoporosis due to vitamin D deficiency or hyperparathyroidism , for example. An oestrogen deficiency can be detected by determining the sex hormones, such as oestradiol and FSH , especially in postmenopausal women.

In the case of hyperparathyroidism , elevated serum calcium levels and elevated PTH levels are characteristic. Imaging , such as an ultrasound examination or scintigraphy of the parathyroid glands, may be required to identify an enlarged or adenomatous parathyroid gland. In advanced cases, X-rays may show typical osteolytic changes, so-called "brown tumours".

The therapy depends on the underlying cause. In the case of hormonal osteoporosis , the focus is on preventing and treating bone loss. This can be achieved through hormone replacement therapy with oestrogens or selective oestrogen receptor modulators (SERMs). In addition, bisphosphonates or denosumab are often used to inhibit osteoclast activity. An adequate supply of calcium and vitamin D is essential. Regular physical activity, especially strength training, can slow down bone loss and improve muscle function.

Hyperparathyroidism is often treated surgically, especially in cases of primary disease caused by a parathyroid adenoma. In mild cases or if surgery is not possible, conservative measures such as optimising the vitamin D and calcium balance and administering calcimimetics can be used to reduce the PTH level.

High blood pressure and electrolyte disorders

High blood pressure and electrolyte imbalances are common symptoms that can indicate endocrine disorders such as aldosterone excess (Conn's syndrome) or cortisol overproduction (Cushing's syndrome). Both disorders affect the hormonal regulation of fluid and electrolyte balance and have profound effects on the cardiovascular system.

Conn's syndrome , also known as primary hyperaldosteronism, is characterised by excessive production of the hormone aldosterone in the adrenal cortex. Aldosterone promotes the reabsorption of sodium and water as well as the excretion of potassium in the kidneys. An excess leads to increased sodium and water retention, which results in hypertension (high blood pressure). At the same time, increased potassium is excreted, causing hypokalaemia. This electrolyte disturbance can lead to symptoms such as muscle weakness , fatigue, cardiac arrhythmia and, in severe cases, to metabolic alkalosis.

Hypertension in Conn's syndrome is often resistant to treatment and occurs at a young age, which should raise suspicion of this cause.

The diagnosis of Conn's syndrome includes measurement of the aldosterone -renin quotient (ARQ), as an elevated ARQ is characteristic of this disease. Further tests, such as the saline load test or the determination of serum potassium, can confirm the diagnosis. Imaging procedures such as computed tomography (CT) or magnetic resonance imaging (MRI) of the adrenal glands are used to identify adenomas or hyperplasia . Selective adrenal vein catheterisation may be necessary to differentiate between unilateral and bilateral aldosterone production.

Cushing's syndrome is characterised by excessive production of cortisol , which is caused either endogenously, e.g. by an adrenal adenoma or pituitary disease (Cushing's disease), or exogenously, e.g. by long-term use of glucocorticoids. Cortisol has a mineralocorticoid effect and can also lead to high blood pressure by increasing the effect of aldosterone in the renin-angiotensin-aldosterone system. In addition, cortisol influences glucose and protein metabolism, which can lead to further symptoms such as weight gain , central fat distribution, muscle weakness and diabetic metabolic conditions. Electrolyte disorders such as hypokalaemia also occur here due to increased potassium excretion.

The diagnosis of Cushing's syndrome includes the measurement of morning serum cortisol, free cortisol in the 24-hour urine collection and the dexamethasone inhibition test. An elevated cortisol level despite the inhibition test speaks in favour of endogenous Cushing's syndrome . To localise the cause, additional tests such as ACTH measurements, a CRH stimulation test or imaging procedures such as MRI of the pituitary gland or CT of the adrenal glands are performed.

The treatment of these disorders depends on the underlying cause. In Conn's syndrome , an adenoma is usually removed surgically, while in the case of bilateral hyperplasia, drug therapies, e.g. with aldosterone antagonists such as spironolactone or eplerenone, are used. In Cushing's syndrome , surgical removal of the hormone-producing tumour, e.g. an adrenal cortex lesion or a pituitary adenoma, is the primary treatment option. In the case of exogenous Cushing's syndrome, a gradual reduction in the glucocorticoid dose is necessary.

Early diagnosis and treatment are crucial, as untreated high blood pressure and electrolyte imbalances can cause serious complications such as cardiovascular disease, kidney damage and metabolic derailment. Interdisciplinary collaboration between endocrinology, nephrology and cardiology is often necessary to ensure the best care for patients.

Role of genetics and epigenetic factors

Genetic factors play an important role in hormonal disorders. Mutations or polymorphisms in genes responsible for hormone production, metabolism or receptors can lead to endocrine disorders. Examples of this are

Monogenic diseases

Monogenic diseases , which are caused by mutations in specific genes, can trigger rare but serious hormonal disorders. Two well-studied examples are **multiple endocrine neoplasia syndrome (MEN)** and **adrenogenital syndrome (AGS)**. Both diseases show how a single genetic change can have profound effects on hormone balance and the function of endocrine organs.

Multiple endocrine neoplasia syndrome (MEN) comprises a group of genetic diseases caused by mutations in the RET gene (MEN type 2) or, more rarely, in the MEN1 gene (MEN type 1). MEN is characterised by the simultaneous or successive development of tumours in several hormone-producing organs. In MEN type 2, which is caused by an activating mutation in the RET protooncogene, medullary thyroid carcinomas, pheochromocytomas and parathyroid hyperplasia typically occur. Medullary thyroid carcinomas often produce calcitonin , which is used for diagnostic purposes. In pheochromocytoma, the excessive production of catecholamines can lead to high blood pressure and other cardiovascular symptoms. MEN type 1, which is caused by a mutation in the MEN1 gene, often leads to tumours in the pituitary gland , the parathyroid glands and the pancreas. The clinical manifestations range from hypercalcaemia due to primary hyperparathyroidism to hormone-producing tumours, such as insulin-producing insulinomas or gastrin-producing gastrinomas.

Adrenogenital syndrome (AGS) is a group of autosomal recessive disorders caused by mutations in genes that code for enzymes involved in steroid synthesis in the adrenal cortex. The most common form of AGS results from a mutation in the CYP21A2 gene, which codes for 21-hydroxylase. This enzyme defect leads to reduced cortisol and aldosterone levels and a compensatory increase in ACTH, which causes an overproduction of precursor steroids, particularly androgens. Clinically, the classic form of AGS often manifests itself in newborns with salt wasting crises, pseudohyperandrogenism or abnormal genital development in female patients. In the non-classical, milder form, symptoms such as hirsutism , cycle disorders or infertility may only occur later in life.

The diagnosis of monogenic hormone disorders involves a combination of clinical observations, biochemical tests and genetic analyses. In MEN syndrome, the mutation in the RET or MEN1 gene is detected by genetic testing, which also enables early identification of asymptomatic carriers. Regular screening examinations such as calcitonin measurement or imaging of the adrenal glands and parathyroid glands are essential in order to detect tumours at an early stage. In AGS , the diagnosis is made by measuring 17-hydroxyprogesterone in the serum, supplemented by genetic tests to identify the specific enzyme defect.

The therapy depends on the specific disease. In MEN syndrome, surgical removal of affected tumours is the most important treatment measure. Prophylactic thyroidectomy is often recommended for MEN type 2 in order to prevent medullary thyroid carcinoma . In AGS , lifelong substitution of glucocorticoids is necessary to suppress ACTH overproduction and control androgen excess . In the classic form, mineralocorticoid substitution is also required to compensate for salt loss.

Early diagnosis and treatment are crucial to prevent complications and improve the quality of life of those affected. Genetic tests also offer the opportunity to examine relatives, offer genetic counselling and initiate preventative measures. Monogenic diseases such as MEN and AGS underline the importance of genetic diagnostics in endocrinology and personalised medicine.

Polygenic influences

Polygenic influences play a central role in the development of common hormonal diseases such as type 2 diabetes mellitus and thyroid disorders. These diseases are multifactorial and result from a complex interplay of genetic predispositions and environmental factors. In contrast to monogenic diseases, in which a mutation in a single gene triggers the disease, polygenic diseases are based on the involvement of many genetic variants, each of which has a small effect on the risk of the disease, but in combination with other factors can significantly increase the likelihood of developing the disease.

Polygenic influences are particularly well documented in **type 2 diabetes mellitus**. Genetic variants in genes such as TCF7L2, FTO, PPARG and KCNJ11 contribute to the increased risk by influencing processes such as insulin secretion, insulin resistance and glucose metabolism . However, genetic predisposition only explains part of the risk, as environmental factors such as an unhealthy diet, lack of exercise, obesity and chronic stress also contribute significantly. The interaction between genetic factors and environmental conditions means that the disease often only manifests itself later in life when the cumulative effects of the risk factors exceed a threshold. Modern approaches such as Genome-Wide Association Studies (GWAS) have identified numerous genetic variants associated with type 2 diabetes. These findings enable personalised medicine in which genetic risk profiles can be used for preventive strategies and therapeutic decisions.

Thyroid diseases, such as **Hashimoto's autoimmune thyroiditis** or **Graves' disease** , are also frequently characterised by polygenic influences. Genetic variants in immune regulation genes, such as HLA-DR3, PTPN22 and CTLA4, increase susceptibility to these autoimmune diseases . They lead to dysregulation of the immune system, which causes inflammation and destruction of thyroid tissue (in Hashimoto's disease) or overproduction of thyroid hormones (in Graves' disease). Environmental factors such as iodine deficiency or excess, smoking, stress and infections can act as triggers or intensifiers of these processes. Women are affected significantly more frequently than men due to hormonal influences and genetic predispositions.

The diagnosis of diseases with polygenic influences combines clinical, biochemical and genetic approaches. For type 2 diabetes , this includes measuring blood glucose and HbA1c levels as well as recording the individual risk profile based on medical history, body weight and lifestyle factors. For thyroid diseases, thyroid function (TSH, fT3, fT4) and specific autoantibodies (e.g. TPO-AK, TRAK) are determined in order to identify autoimmune processes at . Genetic tests can be helpful in research or for specific questions, such as risk assessment in the case of a family history.

The therapeutic approaches take into account both the genetic predisposition and the modifiable environmental factors. For type 2 diabetes , lifestyle changes such as a balanced diet, regular physical activity and weight reduction are the main focus. Drug therapies, such as metformin or SGLT2 inhibitors , are supplemented depending on the individual metabolic situation. In the case of thyroid disorders, treatments are aimed at normalising thyroid function, for example by substituting L-thyroxine for Hashimoto's or thyreostatics and, in severe cases, surgical measures for Graves' disease .

To summarise, polygenic influences show that many hormonal diseases are not attributable to individual genetic mutations, but are caused by the interaction of numerous genetic and environmental factors. These findings enable a holistic approach to prevention and therapy that takes genetic predispositions and lifestyle factors into account in equal measure. Advances in genomics and personalised medicine offer the potential to further improve disease management in the future.

Epigenetic factors

Epigenetic factors , such as DNA methylation , histone modifications and the effect of non-coding RNAs, play a decisive role in the regulation of hormone-relevant genes and thus in the development and function of the endocrine system. These modifications influence whether and how genes are expressed without altering the underlying DNA sequence. As epigenetic patterns can be influenced by environmental factors such as diet, stress, toxins or even lifestyle, they represent an interface between genetics and the environment, which is particularly important in hormonal disorders with a late onset, such as insulin resistance or hormone-dependent cancers

DNA methylation is a common form of epigenetic regulation in which methyl groups are attached to the DNA bases, in particular to cytosine within CpG islands. This modification usually leads to a down-regulation of gene expression. In hormone-relevant genes, deviating methylation can have far-reaching consequences. For example, a hypermethylated promoter region in insulin-regulating genes, such as the insulin receptor gene (INSR), can impair insulin sensitivity and thus contribute to the development of insulin resistance , a precursor to type 2 diabetes . Environmental factors such as a high-calorie diet or lack of exercise can promote these epigenetic changes and thus increase the risk of metabolic diseases.

Histone modifications such as acetylation , methylation or phosphorylation change the structure of the chromatin fibres and thereby influence the accessibility of the DNA for the transcription machinery. Increased acetylation of the histones leads to a loosening of the chromatin and promotes gene expression, while histone methylation can have either an activating or repressive effect, depending on the position of the modification. In hormone-dependent cancers such as breast or prostate cancer , abnormal histone modifications can alter the expression of genes involved in cell growth and differentiation. For example, tumour suppressor genes are downregulated, while oncogenes are activated, which promotes tumour growth.

Epigenetic changes are often reversible, which makes them a promising target for therapeutic intervention. In cancer treatment, drugs such as DNA methyltransferase inhibitors (e.g. acacitidine) and histone deacetylase inhibitors (e.g. vorinostat) are already being used to normalise epigenetic patterns. In future, these approaches could also be used for other hormonal disorders, for example by reactivating silenced genes in metabolic disorders.

A key aspect of epigenetic modifications is their transferability to subsequent generations. Studies show that epigenetic patterns influenced by environmental factors can be partially inherited during germ cell development. This means that a person's diet, stress level or exposure to toxins could influence the health of their offspring. This mechanism, known as transgenerational epigenetics, could explain the increasing prevalence of hormonal disorders in modern societies.

Research into epigenetic factors opens up new perspectives for the prevention and treatment of hormonal disorders. Targeted lifestyle interventions, such as a balanced diet, stress reduction and the avoidance of toxic substances, could positively influence epigenetic changes and reduce the risk of diseases such as insulin resistance or hormone-dependent cancers. In the future, epigenetic markers could also serve as diagnostic tools to assess the individual risk of certain hormonal disorders and develop personalised prevention or therapy approaches.

Types of hormones in therapy

In medical therapy, hormones are used to balance hormonal imbalances, modulate physiological processes or treat specific diseases. The types of hormones used in therapy can be divided into different categories, depending on their chemical structure and function.

Steroid hormones

Steroid hormones are synthesised from cholesterol and are characterised by their lipophilic structure, which allows them to pass through cell membranes and bind intracellularly to receptors .

Oestrogen and progesterone

Oestrogen and progesterone are essential sex hormones that play a central role in the female body and are used in various medical contexts. They are frequently used in hormone replacement therapy (HRT), in oral contraceptives and in fertility medicine to regulate hormonal processes and treat certain conditions.

In **hormone replacement therapy (HRT)**, oestrogen and progesterone are used to alleviate the symptoms of the menopause caused by the natural decline in hormone production in the ovaries. Typical symptoms include hot flushes, sleep disorders, vaginal dryness and mood swings. Oestrogen helps to reduce these symptoms by balancing hormone levels and mitigating the changes caused by the hormone deficiency . Progesterone is often added to minimise the risk of endometrial hyperplasia that can result from oestrogen alone. In addition, hormone replacement therapy has a positive effect on bone health, as oestrogen inhibits bone resorption and thus reduces the risk of osteoporosis and fractures. Despite these benefits, hormone replacement therapy must be carefully considered as it can be associated with risks such as an increased risk of breast cancer and thrombosis . The choice of hormone preparations, dosages and the duration of therapy should be individually adapted to the patient's needs and health risks.

The main components of **oral contraceptives** are oestrogen and progesterone , which are used in combination or as progestogen-only preparations. Combined oral contraceptives work by inhibiting ovulation, thickening the cervical mucus and changing the lining of the uterus, which makes fertilisation and implantation more difficult. These preparations not only offer reliable protection against unwanted pregnancies, but can also alleviate hormonal complaints such as dysmenorrhoea, acne or premenstrual symptoms. Progestogen-only preparations, such as the mini-pill, are an alternative for women who cannot tolerate oestrogens or for whom oestrogens are contraindicated for health reasons, for example if there is an increased risk of thrombosis .

In fertility medicine , oestrogen and progesterone are used specifically to regulate the menstrual cycle and prepare the uterus for a possible pregnancy. Oestrogen helps to build up the lining of the uterus (endometrium), while progesterone stabilises the lining after ovulation and prepares it for the implantation of a fertilised egg. In assisted reproductive technologies such as in vitro fertilisation (IVF), progesterone is often supplemented in the luteal phase in order to optimally prepare the endometrium for embryo implantation and support an early pregnancy. In women with hormonal disorders that affect the menstrual cycle, the administration of these hormones can increase the chances of a successful pregnancy.

In addition to these applications, oestrogen and progesterone also play a role in other medical areas. For example, they are used in the treatment of hormone-dependent diseases such as endometriosis or polycystic ovary syndrome (PCOS) to regulate hormone levels and alleviate symptoms.

Overall, oestrogen and progesterone are indispensable hormones in gynaecology and endocrinology. However, their versatile use requires careful consideration of the benefits and risks, as they can have different side effects or long-term consequences depending on the patient and indication. Advances in personalised medicine make it possible to tailor therapies ever more precisely to the individual needs and health profiles of women.

Testosterone

Testosterone is the primary male sex hormone that plays an important role in physical and mental health in both men and women. In medical practice, testosterone is primarily used in the treatment of male hypogonadism and in hormone replacement therapy for transgender men.

In **hypogonadism** , a condition in which the testicles do not produce enough testosterone , a lack of this hormone can lead to a variety of symptoms, including reduced muscle mass, reduced bone density, loss of libido, erectile dysfunction, fatigue and depressive moods . The causes of hypogonadism can be primary (e.g. due to testicular insufficiency) or secondary (e.g. due to disorders of the hypothalamic-pituitary axis). The diagnosis is made by measuring the total testosterone in the serum, supplemented by the determination of LH and FSH , in order to differentiate the cause.

Testosterone replacement therapy (TRT) is the standard treatment for men with clinically relevant testosterone deficiency. The aim of the therapy is to bring the serum levels of testosterone into the normal physiological range and to alleviate the symptoms of the deficiency. Testosterone is administered in various forms, including transdermal gels, patches, intramuscular injections, subcutaneous implants and oral preparations. The choice of preparation depends on the patient's individual preferences and the desired release kinetics. TRT can increase muscle mass and strength, improve libido and sexual function, increase bone density and have positive effects on mood and energy levels. However, regular monitoring is essential as the therapy carries risks, including a possible increase in haematocrit, worsening of obstructive sleep apnoea and potentially negative effects on the prostate.

Testosterone is also a central component of **hormone replacement therapy for transgender men**. In this context, testosterone is used to promote the development of male secondary sexual characteristics, including a deeper voice, beard growth, increased body hair and an increase in muscle mass. At the same time, it suppresses menstruation and leads to a long-term change in body fat distribution towards a male pattern. The therapy is usually carried out using transdermal gels or intramuscular injections, whereby the dosage is individually adjusted to achieve serum testosterone levels in the male reference range at. Long-term use requires careful monitoring to minimise possible side effects such as dyslipidaemia, polyglobulia or cardiovascular risks.

In addition, testosterone has significance in other medical contexts. In older men with age-related hypogonadism, often referred to as "late-onset hypogonadism", TRT is the subject of controversial debate. While some studies show an improvement in quality of life and physical function, the long-term safety of this therapy, particularly with regard to cardiovascular and oncological risks, has not yet been conclusively clarified.

To summarise, testosterone is an essential hormone whose therapeutic use requires targeted diagnostics and careful monitoring. While treatment for hypogonadism or in transgender medicine can offer significant benefits, an individual risk-benefit assessment is crucial to optimise therapy and minimise potential side effects . Advances in endocrinology and personalised medicine are helping to further improve the efficacy and safety of testosterone therapy.

Corticosteroids (e.g. cortisol , prednisone)

Corticosteroids, such as cortisol and synthetic preparations such as prednisone, are potent steroid hormones , which are used in the treatment of numerous inflammatory and autoimmune diseases. They work by inhibiting the immune response and reducing inflammatory processes by suppressing the expression of pro-inflammatory genes and promoting anti-inflammatory proteins. These properties make them indispensable in the treatment of diseases such as rheumatoid arthritis, asthma, lupus erythematosus and inflammatory bowel disease. In transplant medicine, corticosteroids prevent organ rejection, while in endocrinological disorders such as Addison's disease they replace the lack of natural cortisol production. Despite their effectiveness, long-term or high-dose use harbours risks such as weight gain , high blood pressure , osteoporosis , diabetes , muscle weakness and susceptibility to infection. Psychological changes and suppression of the hypothalamic-pituitary-adrenal axis can also occur, which is why it is necessary to phase out the therapy. Modern synthetic corticosteroids enable more precise application through different strengths and forms of administration, which can reduce systemic side effects . Research is striving for more selective substances in order to further optimise the balance between effectiveness and risk of side effects. Corticosteroids remain essential therapeutics, but require careful customisation to individual needs to ensure maximum benefit with minimum risk.

Peptide hormones

Peptide hormones consist of chains of amino acids and are water-soluble. They bind to membrane receptors and activate intracellular signalling pathways.

Insulin

Insulin is a vital hormone that plays a central role in the treatment of diabetes mellitus. It is used to regulate blood sugar levels and thus stabilise the glucose balance in the body. Insulin promotes the uptake of glucose into the cells and lowers blood sugar by modulating the storage of glucose in the liver as well as fat and protein metabolism. In therapy, insulin is administered in various forms that are tailored to the individual needs of the patient. Short-acting insulins are used before meals to control postprandial blood glucose peaks, while long-acting insulins ensure a constant basal effect over several hours or throughout the day. Modern insulins are often based on genetically engineered, human-identical molecules that enable precise control and dosing while minimising the risk of side effects , such as hypoglycaemia. These further developments not only improve blood glucose control, but also the quality of life of patients, as they enable more individualised and flexible therapy . Insulin therefore remains indispensable in the treatment of type 1 diabetes and advanced stages of type 2 diabetes.

Growth hormones (somatropin)

Growth hormones (somatropin) are essential peptide hormones that are used in the treatment of children with growth hormone deficiency and adults with pituitary dysfunction. They play a central role in the regulation of growth and metabolism by promoting cell proliferation, differentiation and regeneration. In children with growth hormone deficiency, the hormone is used to stimulate longitudinal growth and enable normal physical development. In adults suffering from growth hormone deficiency due to pituitary dysfunction, it is used to improve body composition, increase muscle mass and reduce fatty tissue. Growth hormone also supports protein synthesis by promoting the synthesis of amino acids into proteins and helps to maintain bone density and regulate energy metabolism. Modern therapies use genetically engineered, recombinant growth hormones that are biologically identical to the human hormone, which enables precise and effective treatment. However, their use requires careful monitoring, as side effects such as joint pain, oedema or insulin resistance can occur. Growth hormones are an indispensable part of the treatment of growth hormone deficiency and offer affected patients a significantly improved quality of life and physical function.

Glucagon

Glucagon is a vital hormone that is used in emergency medicine to treat hypoglycaemic crises. It works by stimulating the release of glucose from the liver's glycogen stores, which rapidly increases blood glucose levels. Glucagon binds to specific receptors on liver cells and activates glycogenolysis, in which stored glycogen is converted into glucose and released into the blood. At the same time, it promotes gluconeogenesis, i.e. the new synthesis of glucose from non-carbohydrate precursors, which supports a sustained increase in blood sugar levels. It is typically administered as an intramuscular or subcutaneous injection and is particularly effective in patients with severe hypoglycaemia who are no longer able to ingest carbohydrates orally. Glucagon is an essential therapeutic option, especially for insulin-treated diabetics, and can rapidly resolve life-threatening conditions. Modern dosage forms, such as pre-filled syringes or nasal applications, make it easier to use and help to make treatment safe and effective, even for non-professionals.

Erythropoietin (EPO)

The peptide hormone erythropoietin (EPO) is used to treat anaemia, particularly in patients with chronic renal insufficiency. Erythropoietin is produced physiologically in the kidneys and plays a central role in the regulation of erythropoiesis by stimulating the formation and maturation of red blood cells in the bone marrow. In chronic renal insufficiency, erythropoietin production is often reduced, leading to anaemia, which manifests itself as fatigue, weakness and reduced performance. The therapeutic administration of recombinant erythropoietin corrects the hormone deficiency, increases the haemoglobin concentration and improves the oxygen supply to the tissue. Erythropoietin is administered subcutaneously or intravenously and is also useful for other causes of anaemia, such as chemotherapy-induced anaemia. Therapy requires careful monitoring as excessive increases in haemoglobin are associated with an increased risk of thromboembolic events and hypertension. Erythropoietin is an essential component of modern anaemia treatment and contributes significantly to improving the quality of life of affected patients.

Thyroid hormones

Thyroid hormones , in particular thyroxine (T4) and triiodothyronine (T3), play a central role in the metabolism .

Levothyroxine (synthetic T4)

Levothyroxine , a synthetic analogue of the thyroid hormone thyroxine (T4), is the standard medication for the treatment of hypothyroidism . It replaces or supplements the inadequate production of thyroid hormones and thus restores normal thyroid function. After oral administration, levothyroxine is converted in the body to triiodothyronine (T3), the biologically active form of the hormone that exerts metabolic and regulatory effects on the target tissues.

Due to its long half-life of around seven days, levothyroxine is well suited to ensuring stable hormone levels in the blood. The dosage is adjusted individually based on the TSH values and the free T4 level, which are monitored regularly to avoid under- or overdosing. The medication is usually taken in the morning on an empty stomach, as absorption can be impaired by food or certain medications.

It is mainly used to treat primary hypothyroidism caused by diseases such as Hashimoto's thyroiditis or following surgical removal of the thyroid gland . It is also used for secondary hypothyroidism when the pituitary gland or the hypothalamus are affected. At the correct dosage, levothyroxine normalises metabolic functions, alleviates symptoms such as tiredness, weight gain and sensitivity to cold and significantly improves the patient's quality of life. The therapy is considered safe and well tolerated, but requires long-term, often lifelong use.

Liothyronine (synthetic T3)

Liothyronine, a synthetic analogue of the thyroid hormone triiodothyronine (T3), is used in certain cases to treat thyroid disorders. Compared to levothyroxine (T4), liothyronine has a significantly shorter half-life of around 24 hours, which requires more frequent intake and can lead to greater fluctuations in hormone levels .

Due to these properties, liothyronine is used less frequently as monotherapy. It is mainly used in patients who continue to show symptoms of hypothyroidism despite optimal doses of levothyroxine , as T3 is the active form of the hormone that acts directly on the target tissues. In such cases, it is often used in combination therapies with T4 in order to achieve a more balanced supply of thyroid hormones .

Liothyronine is also used in special clinical situations, for example in myxoedema coma, a rare, life-threatening complication of hypothyroidism . In such emergencies, the rapid effect of T3 enables a rapid improvement in the patient's condition. It can also be used temporarily to normalise hormone levels in patients who are preparing for radioiodine therapy or who require suppressive therapy.

The use of Liothyronine requires careful monitoring, as overdoses can easily lead to symptoms of hyperthyroidism such as palpitations, restlessness or insomnia. Despite its more limited indications, it remains a valuable drug in endocrinology, especially for patients with specific therapeutic requirements.

Antithyroid drugs

Antithyroid drugs such as methimazole and propylthiouracil are essential drugs for the treatment of hyperthyroidism . They work by inhibiting thyroid hormone production by blocking the enzyme thyroperoxidase, which is involved in the iodination of tyrosine residues and the synthesis of T3 and T4. Propylthiouracil has the additional ability to inhibit the peripheral conversion of T4 to T3, which makes it particularly useful in acute situations such as thyrotoxic crisis.

These drugs are mainly used in hyperthyroidism diseases such as Graves' disease to control the overproduction of thyroid hormones . They are often used as an initial treatment option, particularly in patients who are not suitable for radioiodine therapy or surgical treatment, or as preparation for these procedures. The duration of treatment is usually 12 to 18 months, with regular thyroid function checks required to adjust the dosage and prevent the development of hypothyroidism .

Antithyroid drugs are generally well tolerated, but can cause side effects such as skin rashes, joint pain or gastrointestinal complaints. More serious complications, such as agranulocytosis (severe reduction of white blood cells) or hepatotoxicity, are rare but require immediate discontinuation of therapy and medical intervention. Propylthiouracil is usually only preferred when methimazole is not suitable, for example during the first trimester of pregnancy, due to its higher risk of liver damage.

Antithyroid drugs remain a central component in the treatment of hyperthyroidism , offer effective control of the disease and make it possible to stabilise thyroid function without invasive measures. However, their use requires careful monitoring in order to recognise side effects at an early stage and to make the therapy safe and effective.

Synthetic and bioidentical hormones

The further development of hormone replacement therapy has led to a distinction being made between synthetic and bioidentical hormones.

Synthetic hormones

Synthetic hormones are chemically produced compounds that are either identical to natural hormones or have been modified to improve their pharmacological properties. They are widely used in medicine, for example in contraception, hormone replacement therapy or the treatment of hormone-dependent diseases. A well-known example is ethinylestradiol, a modified oestrogen , which is contained in many oral contraceptives . The introduction of an ethinyl group into the molecular structure increases stability against metabolic degradation and improves bioavailability, so that a lower dose is required to achieve effective hormone level control.

Such chemical modifications can also give synthetic hormones a longer duration of action, which can extend treatment intervals and improve compliance. For example, long-acting insulin analogues or depot preparations of synthetic progestins are used in clinical practice to ensure a continuous and stable effect. At the same time, synthetic hormones allow specific receptors to be influenced in a targeted manner, whereby certain effects can be enhanced or undesirable effects minimised.

However, synthetic hormones can also cause specific side effects resulting from their modified structure. Ethinylestradiol, for example, increases the risk of thrombosis in some women due to its influence on coagulation factor metabolism. Similar challenges exist with other synthetic hormones, whose long-term effects on the body can vary from individual to individual.

The development of synthetic hormones has significantly advanced modern medicine, as it allows hormones to be precisely customised to therapeutic needs. Nevertheless, their use requires careful consideration of benefits and risks as well as customised dosing to ensure effective and safe treatment. Research is continuously working on improving synthetic hormones in order to increase their effectiveness and further minimise potential side effects .

Bioidentical hormones

Bioidentical hormones are synthetically produced hormones whose molecular structure is identical to the body's own hormones. They are usually synthesised from plant precursors such as diosgenin, which is obtained from yams or soya, and chemically converted into substances such as oestrogen , progesterone or testosterone . Due to their identical structure, they can bind to the natural hormone receptors and trigger physiological effects that are similar to the body's own hormone.

Proponents of bioidentical hormones emphasise that these substances are better tolerated and more natural in their effect, as they are metabolised in the same way as the body's own hormones. They are often used in hormone replacement therapy (HRT) in menopausal women to alleviate symptoms such as hot flushes, sleep disorders and mood swings, as well as in the treatment of hormone deficiencies in men or endocrine disorders.

Despite their advantages, there are challenges when using bioidentical hormones. One major point of criticism is the lack of standardisation, particularly in the case of individually manufactured formulations that are prepared in pharmacies (so-called "compounding pharmacies"). These preparations are not always subject to the same strict regulatory requirements as conventional hormone preparations, which can lead to fluctuations in dosage and potential safety risks. In addition, bioidentical hormones are often more expensive than synthetic alternatives, which can limit availability and access.

The scientific evidence clearly demonstrating the advantages of bioidentical hormones over synthetic hormones is limited. Nevertheless, they are a valuable option for patients who prefer nature-identical hormone therapy or experience side effects with conventional preparations. Careful monitoring of therapy and individual adjustment of dosage are essential to maximise efficacy and minimise risks. Further research into bioidentical hormones could help to better understand their safety and effectiveness and establish standardised treatment options.

Importance of hormones in therapy

The diversity of hormones in therapy opens up numerous possibilities for the targeted treatment of a wide range of clinical pictures, as they can intervene in almost all of the body's central regulatory processes. Steroid hormones , such as oestrogen , progesterone , testosterone and glucocorticoids, are indispensable components of modern medicine and are widely used in hormone replacement therapy, oncology and immunomodulation. They are used, for example, to alleviate menopausal symptoms such as hot flushes and osteoporosis , to remedy the symptoms of testosterone deficiency or to suppress the immune response in inflammatory and autoimmune diseases such as rheumatoid arthritis or asthma. Their broad spectrum of action makes them indispensable in many areas, but requires precise dosing and monitoring, as they can also be associated with side effects such as an increased risk of thrombosis , metabolic disorders or suppression of the body's own hormone production systems.

Peptide hormones , such as insulin , glucagon or erythropoietin, are essential in the regulation of metabolic processes and the support of physiological functions. Insulin plays a central role in the treatment of diabetes mellitus, where it normalises glucose metabolism and prevents life-threatening complications such as ketoacidosis. Glucagon is used in emergency situations to treat severe hypoglycaemia, while erythropoietin is used in anaemia, particularly chronic renal failure, to promote erythrocyte formation in the bone marrow. These hormones have the potential to be life-saving and are examples of the precise control of the body's own processes through hormonal interventions.

Thyroid hormones , such as levothyroxine and liothyronine, are indispensable in endocrinology, as they form the basis for the treatment of hypothyroidism and hyperthyroidism . In hypothyroidism, levothyroxine replaces the missing T4 and is converted to T3 in the body, which normalises the metabolism and the patient's quality of life. In special situations, such as acute thyroid crises or special hormonal requirements, the fast-acting liothyronine is also used. The regulation of thyroid hormone levels is crucial, as both a deficiency and an excess can have serious effects on the entire organism.

Synthetic hormones and bioidentical hormones significantly expand the therapeutic spectrum by enabling more individualised treatment. Synthetic hormones, such as ethinylestradiol in contraceptive pills, offer advantages through chemical modifications such as improved bioavailability, a longer duration of action or targeted receptor binding, which increases their effectiveness. Bioidentical hormones , on the other hand, which are structurally identical to the body's own hormones, are often perceived as more natural and better tolerated, as they undergo the same metabolic pathways as endogenous hormones. Their production from plant precursors, such as diosgenin from yam roots, enables precise customisation to the physiological needs of the patient. Nevertheless, bioidentical hormones are often more expensive and not always standardised, which requires careful consideration when using them.

The selection of the appropriate hormone and its form of administration is always based on the specific diagnosis, the individual needs of the patient and a thorough risk-benefit assessment. Hormonal preparations can be administered orally, subcutaneously, intravenously, transdermally or intramuscularly, depending on the desired duration of action, site of action and tolerability. Advances in medical research and development have continuously improved the safety and efficacy of hormonal therapies. This includes the development of long-acting depot preparations, the optimisation of combination preparations and the introduction of new administration systems that enable more individualised and convenient therapy.

Hormone therapy is an indispensable part of modern medicine, as it enables precise control of bodily processes and can effectively treat a variety of diseases. Its wide range of applications, from endocrinology and oncology to metabolic medicine, demonstrate its enormous potential. Advances in research and the further development of synthetic and bioidentical hormones will continue to help expand treatment options and further improve patients' quality of life in the future.

Part II: Application of hormone therapies

Hormone therapy in gynaecology

Hormone therapy (HT) plays a central role in gynaecological practice, particularly in the treatment of symptoms associated with hormonal changes such as the menopause . It involves the targeted use of hormones to compensate for endocrine deficiencies or to modulate physiological processes. The most common form of HT in gynaecology is hormone replacement therapy (HRT), which is primarily used to treat menopausal and perimenopausal symptoms.

Menopause and perimenopausal symptoms

The menopause , defined as the permanent cessation of menstruation due to the cessation of ovarian function, is accompanied by a significant hormonal change. The associated drop in oestrogen and progesterone levels can cause a variety of symptoms that can significantly affect the well-being and quality of life of the women affected.

Typical symptoms are

- **Vasomotor complaints**: Hot flushes and night sweats, which are the most common reasons for seeking hormone replacement therapy.

- **Psychological symptoms**: sleep disorders, irritability, depressive moods and concentration problems.
- **Urogenital complaints**: Vaginal dryness, dyspareunia and frequent urinary tract infections due to atrophic changes in the mucous membrane.
- **Bone and muscle complaints**: Increased bone resorption for hormone replacement therapy leads to a risk of osteoporosis and fractures.
- **Cardiovascular symptoms**: changes in lipid metabolism and increased cardiovascular risks.

The perimenopausal phase, the transition phase to the menopause , is particularly characterised by hormonal fluctuations that can exacerbate these symptoms.

Hormone replacement therapy (HRT): Indications, benefits and risks

Hormone replacement therapy (HRT) is a central component of the treatment of menopausal symptoms and is used in particular to alleviate symptoms caused by the decline in oestrogen production during the menopause . The most important indications include symptom relief for vasomotor complaints such as hot flushes and night sweats as well as psychological symptoms such as sleep disorders, irritability and depression. These symptoms can have a considerable impact on quality of life, meaning that targeted therapy can significantly improve the well-being of many women.

Another important indication for hormone replacement therapy is the treatment of urogenital atrophy. The oestrogen deficiency during the menopause often leads to atrophic changes in the vaginal and urethral mucous membranes, which can cause symptoms such as vaginal dryness, dyspareunia and recurrent urinary tract infections. In such cases, hormone replacement therapy can be used both locally and systemically, with local application being preferred in order to minimise systemic risks.

The prevention of osteoporosis is another important indication. After the menopause , the risk of bone loss and associated fractures increases, particularly in the spine and hips. Hormone replacement therapy has proven to be an effective measure for reducing this risk, as it has a positive effect on bone metabolism and maintains bone density. Hormone replacement therapy is also indicated for women with primary ovarian insufficiency, to compensate for hormonal deficiencies, which can lead not only to menopausal symptoms but also to long-term health risks.

The benefits of hormone replacement therapy lie primarily in the improvement in quality of life. The alleviation of symptoms such as hot flushes, sleep disorders and psychological complaints enables the women affected to cope better with their everyday lives. In addition, hormone replacement therapy contributes to bone health by significantly reducing the risk of osteoporotic fractures. Another potential benefit is protection against cardiovascular disease, especially if hormone replacement therapy is initiated early in the perimenopause. However, these protective effects on the cardiovascular system depend on the timing of the initiation of therapy and require further research.

Despite the many benefits, hormone replacement therapy also harbours risks that must be carefully weighed up. Known risks include thromboembolic events such as venous thrombosis and pulmonary embolism, which can occur particularly with systemic hormone replacement therapy. Another potentially increased risk is the development of breast cancer, particularly with prolonged use of combined hormone replacement therapy with oestrogen and progestogen. Women with an intact uterus who do not receive adequate progesterone administration also have an increased risk of endometrial hyperplasia , which in some cases can lead to endometrial cancer. Cardiovascular risks also vary depending on the time and duration of use and must be assessed on an individual basis.

In order to minimise the risks of hormone replacement therapy, certain strategies are of crucial importance. These include using the lowest effective amount of hormone to achieve the desired therapeutic effects while minimising side effects . Where possible, local application should be preferred, for example for urogenital complaints, as this method minimises systemic exposure. In addition, regular evaluation of the risk-benefit ratio is essential in order to customise the therapy and ensure patient safety. Such regular reviews make it possible to recognise potential risks at an early stage and modify the therapy accordingly.

Prevention and treatment of osteoporosis

Osteoporosis is one of the most common and significant complications associated with postmenopausal oestrogen deficiency. The decline in oestrogen production after the menopause leads to accelerated bone loss, as the osteoprotective effects of oestrogens are absent. Oestrogens play a central role in bone metabolism by regulating the balance between bone formation and bone resorption. In their absence, the activity of osteoclasts , which are responsible for the breakdown of bone tissue, is increased, while the activity of osteoblasts , which are responsible for bone formation, cannot be sufficiently compensated. This leads to a decrease in bone density and increased fragility of the skeleton, which significantly increases the risk of fractures, particularly in stress-relevant areas such as the spine and hips.

Hormone replacement therapy is an effective measure to counteract this pathophysiological process. It offers both preventive and therapeutic benefits, especially for women who are at high risk of osteoporotic fractures. The primary mechanism of action of hormone replacement therapy in the prevention of osteoporosis is the inhibition of osteoclast activity by oestrogens . These hormones interact with specific receptors on the bone cells, suppressing the release of cytokines and growth factors that promote osteoclast activity. At the same time, the apoptosis of osteoclasts is promoted and the lifespan of osteoblasts is extended, which leads to a stabilisation of bone metabolism.

The use of oestrogens as part of hormone replacement therapy reduces bone resorption, which not only enables the existing bone density to be maintained, but in many cases also a moderate increase. This has a direct effect on the mechanical stability of the bone and leads to a reduction in the risk of osteoporotic fractures. Hormone replacement therapy has a significant protective effect, especially in the early postmenopause, when bone loss is most pronounced.

In addition to the direct effect on bone metabolism , hormone replacement therapy also has systemic effects that can contribute to the prevention of osteoporosis . For example, it improves calcium absorption in the intestine and reduces renal calcium excretion, which increases the availability of this essential mineral for bone formation. In addition, hormone replacement therapy can modulate inflammatory processes in bone tissue, which also play a role in pathological bone loss.

Despite its effectiveness, the use of hormone replacement therapy to prevent osteoporosis must be carefully considered, as it is associated with specific risks. The decision in favour of hormone replacement therapy should therefore be made on an individual basis, taking into account the patient's general health, her fracture risk and possible contraindications. Regular check-ups are necessary to check the effectiveness of the therapy and to recognise possible side effects at an early stage. Ultimately, hormone replacement therapy is a valuable option for many women to maintain their quality of life and minimise the long-term consequences of osteoporosis .

Alternatives to hormone replacement therapy

Bisphosphonates

Bisphosphonates are an established and effective alternative to hormone replacement therapy (HRT) for the prevention and treatment of osteoporosis , particularly in women for whom HRT is contraindicated or does not want to be used. These drugs have a targeted effect on bone metabolism and are particularly important for postmenopausal osteoporosis and other forms of bone loss.

The mechanism of action of bisphosphonates is based on their ability to selectively adhere to the surface of bone, particularly in areas of high bone remodelling. They are taken up by active osteoclasts and inhibit their function by interfering with cell metabolism. In particular, they block farnesyl pyrophosphate synthase, an enzyme in the mevalonate metabolic pathway that is essential for the function and survival of osteoclasts. This leads to the inhibition of bone resorption without impairing bone formation by osteoblasts , resulting in a stabilisation or increase in bone density.

Areas of application and advantages of bisphosphonates

Bisphosphonates are approved for both the prevention and treatment of osteoporosis . They reduce the risk of vertebral and non-vertebral fractures, including hip fractures, and are highly effective in patients with pre-existing osteoporosis or multiple risk factors. Commonly used agents include alendronate , risedronate , ibandronate and zoledronate .

A major advantage of bisphosphonates is that, unlike hormone replacement therapy, they do not have any oestrogen-dependent side effects such as an increased risk of breast cancer or endometrial cancer. They are also suitable for patients who cannot take hormones due to the risk of thrombosis or embolism.

Application forms and dosage

Bisphosphonates are administered in various forms, including oral tablets (e.g. weekly or monthly) and intravenous infusions (e.g. annually for zoledronate). This flexibility allows the therapy to be customised to the patient's needs and preferences.

Side effects and restrictions

Despite their effectiveness, bisphosphonates are associated with specific side effects . Oral preparations can cause gastrointestinal complaints such as heartburn, nausea and oesophagitis, which is why they must be taken with sufficient water and in an upright position. Long-term use, especially beyond five years, is associated with rare but serious complications such as atypical femoral fractures and osteonecrosis of the jaw (ONJ). These risks require regular re-evaluation of the therapy and possibly therapy breaks (so-called "drug holidays").

Denosumab

Denosumab is a monoclonal antibody that specifically blocks the Receptor Activator of Nuclear Factor κB Ligand (RANKL), an essential signalling pathway that regulates the activity and differentiation of osteoclasts . As a RANKL inhibitor, denosumab has a unique mechanism of action compared to other therapies for the treatment and prevention of osteoporosis . It is used in particular in postmenopausal women at high risk of fracture and represents an effective alternative or supplement to traditional treatments such as bisphosphonates.

Mechanism of action of denosumab

RANKL is a protein that is produced by osteoblasts and their precursor cells and is necessary for the maturation and activation of osteoclasts . Osteoclasts are the cells responsible for bone resorption. Denosumab binds specifically to RANKL and prevents its interaction with the RANK receptor on the osteoclasts. This inhibition reduces the formation, function and lifespan of osteoclasts, which leads to a significant reduction in bone resorption. This leads to an increase in bone density and a reduction in the risk of osteoporotic fractures.

Indications for denosumab

Denosumab is primarily used in postmenopausal osteoporosis , especially in women at high risk of fractures or with intolerance or contraindications to bisphosphonates. It is also used in other conditions associated with increased bone resorption, such as glucocorticoid-induced osteoporosis or in men undergoing hormone-suppressive therapy for prostate cancer .

Advantages of denosumab

Denosumab offers several significant advantages over traditional osteoporosis therapies and represents an attractive option for patients in need of alternative treatment options. One of the most outstanding strengths of denosumab is its efficacy, as it significantly reduces the risk of vertebral, non-vertebral and hip fractures. This comprehensive protection against fractures makes it an effective choice for women with postmenopausal osteoporosis, especially those at high risk of fracture. Another advantage is the convenience of use. Since denosumab is injected subcutaneously and only needs to be administered twice a year, adherence to therapy is made much easier compared to other forms of treatment that require more frequent doses. This is particularly beneficial for older patients who may have difficulty adhering to complex dosing regimes.

An additional feature that distinguishes denosumab from other osteoporosis therapies is its wider applicability in patients with renal impairment. While bisphosphonates are often contraindicated in patients with impaired renal function, denosumab can be used safely as it is not excreted via the kidneys. This expands the treatment options for a patient group that is frequently affected by osteoporosis and has limited treatment options.

Risks of denosumab

Despite its benefits, denosumab is not free from risks and possible side effects , which must be carefully monitored. One common complication is hypocalcaemia, which can occur particularly in patients with limited calcium absorption or vitamin D deficiency. It is therefore essential to ensure adequate supplementation of calcium and vitamin D before starting and during therapy in order to compensate for this deficiency. There is also a slightly increased risk of infections of the skin and soft tissue, such as cellulitis, which must be taken into account when using denosumab.

A rare but potentially serious complication is osteonecrosis of the jaw (ONJ), which can occur in a similar way to bisphosphonates, particularly with prolonged therapy. The development of ONJ requires careful dental monitoring and early intervention in order to avoid serious consequences. Another long-term complication that can occur in rare cases is atypical femoral fractures. These rare fractures require regular monitoring, especially with prolonged use of denosumab .

Restrictions and weaning problems

A special feature of denosumab is the rebound effect after discontinuation of therapy. Discontinuation can lead to a rapid and strong increase in osteoclast activity, which can result in accelerated bone loss and an increased risk of multiple vertebral fractures. It is therefore important to consider an alternative treatment, such as bisphosphonates , to control bone loss after denosumab therapy is discontinued.

Overall, denosumab is an effective and convenient option for the treatment of osteoporosis , particularly in patients with a high risk of fracture or intolerance to other therapies. Its innovative mechanism of action and infrequent injections make it an attractive choice. Nevertheless, its use requires careful monitoring and strategic planning, particularly with regard to possible side effects and management after the end of therapy.

Selective oestrogen receptor modulators (SERMs)

Selective oestrogen receptor modulators (SERMs) are an important alternative in the treatment and prevention of osteoporosis , especially for women who refuse hormone replacement therapy (HRT) or for whom HRT is contraindicated. SERMs are synthetic compounds, which act on oestrogen receptors but show either agonistic or antagonistic effects depending on the tissue. This selective action makes it possible to utilise the positive effects of oestrogens on bone metabolism without increasing the risks associated with oestrogen-dependent diseases such as breast carcinoma or endometrial carcinoma.

SERMs effectively protect against osteoporotic fractures by inhibiting the activity of osteoclasts and reducing bone resorption. Their mechanism of action is based on the fact that they act like oestrogens in bone tissue and reduce the expression of osteoclast-stimulating factors there. As a result, they promote the maintenance or even an increase in bone density and strengthen the mechanical stability of the skeleton. Studies have shown that SERMs such as raloxifene significantly reduce the risk of vertebral fractures, whereby the benefit is particularly pronounced in women with pre-existing osteoporosis .

A key advantage of SERMs compared to hormone replacement therapy is that they do not have a stimulating effect on breast tissue. On the contrary, raloxifene actually lowers the risk of oestrogen receptor-positive breast cancer, making it a preferred choice for women who are at increased risk of breast cancer or have a history of breast cancer. In addition, SERMs do not increase the risk of endometrial hyperplasia or carcinoma, which further improves their safety profiles.

Despite their benefits, SERMs also have side effects and limitations that must be considered when planning therapy. One of the most common side effects is the increased risk of venous thromboembolic events, including deep vein thrombosis and pulmonary embolism. This risk is similar to that observed with hormone replacement therapy and therefore requires careful consideration in patients with a history of such events. Other possible side effects include hot flushes and muscle cramps, which can affect the quality of life of some women.

SERMs are most effective in preventing vertebral fractures and less effective in reducing the risk of hip fractures compared to other therapies such as bisphosphonates or denosumab . They are therefore particularly suitable for postmenopausal women with a moderate fracture risk or for those seeking additional protection against breast cancer .

To summarise, SERMs such as raloxifene are a versatile and safe option in the treatment of osteoporosis, particularly due to their protective effects on bone and their cancer-preventive properties. However, their benefits are greatest with targeted patient selection and taking into account potential risks, particularly with regard to thromboembolic complications. Regular monitoring and customisation of therapy are crucial to ensure the maximum benefit of these drugs.

Vitamin D and calcium

Vitamin D and calcium play a fundamental role in maintaining and promoting bone stability and are essential components of any strategy for the prevention and treatment of osteoporosis . Both nutrients act synergistically to support bone metabolism , maintain bone mineral density and reduce the risk of fractures.

Calcium is the most important mineral that is stored in the bones and ensures their strength and stability. Around 99% of all calcium in the body is found in bones and teeth. Calcium is not only a structural component, but is also essential for numerous physiological processes, such as muscle contraction, blood clotting and the function of enzymes. Insufficient calcium levels in the blood cause the body to mobilise calcium from the bones in order to maintain vital functions, which can lead to bone loss and osteoporosis in the long term.

Vitamin D is also essential as it promotes the absorption of calcium from the intestine and regulates the homeostasis of calcium in the blood. Without sufficient amounts of vitamin D, only a fraction of the calcium ingested through food is effectively absorbed, which can lead to a calcium deficiency and thus to impaired bone health. Vitamin D also helps to stimulate osteoblast activity, which is responsible for bone formation, and inhibits the release of parathyroid hormone (PTH), which in high concentrations promotes bone resorption.

The combined intake of vitamin D and calcium is particularly important in the prevention and treatment of osteoporosis , especially in postmenopausal women, the elderly and people at increased risk of fractures. Studies have shown that regular intake of both nutrients stabilises or even increases bone density and reduces the risk of vertebral and non-vertebral fractures.

A lack of vitamin D , which is widespread worldwide, especially in regions with limited sunlight, can have a significant impact on bone health. Vitamin D is mainly synthesised in the skin under UVB radiation, and only a small amount is absorbed from food. Therefore, vitamin D supplementation is often necessary, especially in older people whose ability to synthesise vitamin D in the skin is reduced.

The recommended daily intake of calcium is between 1000 and 1200 mg, depending on age and gender, while vitamin D intake should be around 800 to 2000 IU per day, especially for at-risk groups. Exceeding these doses should be avoided, however, as excessive calcium intake is associated with an increased risk of kidney stones and excessive vitamin D intake with hypercalcaemia.

To summarise, vitamin D and calcium are essential components for maintaining bone health and preventing osteoporosis . Their synergistic effect ensures that the body is adequately supplied with calcium and that it can be utilised efficiently. Regular intake through a balanced diet, supplemented by dietary supplements if necessary, as well as adequate exposure to sunlight are crucial to ensure the long-term stability and strength of bones.

Hormone therapy in andrology

Hormone therapy in andrology (= speciality that deals with male health, in particular the function and disease of the male reproductive organs, hormonal disorders, reproductive ability and sexual dysfunction), especially testosterone replacement therapy (TRT), plays a central role in the treatment of testosterone deficiency and hypogonadism . Testosterone is the most important male sex hormone and is essential for numerous physiological processes, including sexual health, muscle mass development, bone density and general quality of life. A lack of testosterone, known as hypogonadism, can occur primarily due to testicular dysfunction or secondarily as a result of dysfunction of the hypothalamic-pituitary axis. This condition often leads to symptoms such as decreased libido, erectile dysfunction, fatigue, muscle loss, increased body fat and psychological impairments such as depression and irritability. Bone health can also be affected by a decrease in bone density and an increased risk of osteoporosis .

Testosterone replacement therapy is the standard treatment for symptomatic hypogonadism and is administered in various forms, including intramuscular injections, transdermal gels or patches, subcutaneous implants and oral preparations. It aims to normalise testosterone levels and alleviate the associated symptoms. Studies show that TRT significantly improves libido and sexual function, which has a direct positive impact on the quality of life of the men affected. In addition, TRT affects muscle metabolism by stimulating protein synthesis, which leads to an increase in muscle mass and strength. At the same time, it reduces fat mass, which promotes body composition and metabolic health. The improvement in bone density under TRT can reduce the risk of osteoporotic fractures, especially in men with advanced testosterone deficiency.

The impact of testosterone on cardiovascular health is complex and controversial. While low testosterone levels are associated with metabolic syndrome, insulin resistance and obesity, the question of whether TRT increases or reduces cardiovascular risks remains open. Some studies suggest positive effects on lipid metabolism and endothelial function, while others suggest an increased risk of thromboembolic events or cardiovascular disease. For this reason, a careful individual risk-benefit assessment is required before starting TRT.

TRT is increasingly being discussed in the context of so-called anti-ageing, with older men often receiving testosterone without a clear indication as a means of improving vitality, muscle strength and quality of life. Even though some studies suggest that TRT may have benefits in this group, there is not yet a sufficient scientific basis for widespread use. In addition, risks such as polycythaemia, thromboembolic events or adverse effects on the prostate may predominate, especially with long-term use without a clear medical indication.

Hormone therapy in andrology offers clear benefits in the treatment of testosterone deficiency and hypogonadism , particularly in terms of improving sexual function, muscle mass and quality of life. At the same time, it requires careful medical monitoring in order to minimise possible side effects and identify risks such as cardiovascular complications or prostate diseases at an early stage. The use of testosterone therapy as an anti-ageing measure remains controversial and should be viewed with caution, as comprehensive scientific evidence for its safety and efficacy in this context is still lacking. Careful selection of patients and regular monitoring of therapy are crucial in order to maximise the benefits of TRT and minimise potential risks.

Hormonal treatments in reproductive medicine

Hormonal treatments are a central part of reproductive medicine and are used to diagnose and treat both female and male fertility problems. In women, hormones play a crucial role in stimulating ovulation, regulating the menstrual cycle and optimising the conditions for the implantation of a fertilised egg. In men, hormonal approaches are used to improve sperm production and quality when these are impaired by endocrine disorders.

Stimulating ovulation and regulating the menstrual cycle are essential steps in the treatment of female infertility . In women with irregular or absent ovulation , such as those with polycystic ovary syndrome (PCOS), ovulation inducers such as clomiphene or letrozole are used to promote follicular maturation and trigger ovulation. Gonadotropins, including follicle stimulating hormone (FSH) and luteinising hormone (LH), are often used to support the development of multiple follicles, particularly in assisted reproductive techniques such as in vitro fertilisation (IVF). In IVF, hormonal stimulation is of central importance in order to maximise egg maturation and increase the chances of successful fertilisation. At the same time, hormones such as gonadotropin-releasing hormone (GnRH) analogues or GnRH antagonists are used to suppress the natural cycle and enable precise control of hormone levels . After egg retrieval, progesterone is often administered to support the luteal phase and create optimal conditions for implantation of the fertilised egg.

In addition to stimulating the ovaries, hormonal treatment also plays a key role in preparing the endometrium. Oestrogen and progesterone are often used in combination to prepare the endometrium to receive the embryo. This is particularly important in techniques such as embryo transfer preparation in the cryocycle, where frozen embryos are transferred and synchronisation between the endometrium and the developmental stage of the embryo is essential.

In men with infertility problems caused by hormonal dysfunctions such as hypogonadism or disorders of the hypothalamic-pituitary axis, hormonal therapies are used to promote spermatogenesis. Gonadotropins such as human chorionic gonadotropin (hCG) and recombinant FSH can be used to stimulate testicular function and increase sperm production. These therapies are particularly effective in men with secondary hypogonadism, as they mimic the natural hormonal control cycle. In certain cases, testosterone replacement is also used, but only in men who are not trying to conceive, as exogenous testosterone can suppress sperm production.

Hormonal treatments are also of central importance in the diagnosis and treatment of complex fertility problems. Monitoring hormone levels such as FSH , LH, estradiol, progesterone and anti-Müllerian hormone (AMH) provides valuable information about ovarian reserve, cycle regulation and the causes of infertility . This data enables the individualisation of treatment plans, to maximise the chances of success with assisted reproductive techniques.

In summary, hormonal treatments are an integral part of reproductive medicine , as they optimise the conditions for successful reproduction in both women and men . They enable targeted control of the menstrual cycle , support egg maturation and promote sperm production. Despite their effectiveness, these therapies require careful monitoring in order to avoid side effects such as ovarian hyperstimulation syndrome (OHSS) in women or hormonal imbalances in men. The customisation of hormonal treatments to the specific needs of patients is crucial to the success of reproductive medicine interventions.

Oncology and hormone therapy

Hormone therapy plays a central role in oncology , particularly in the treatment of hormone-dependent tumours such as breast cancer and prostate cancer . These tumour types often exhibit hormonal dependence, with hormones such as oestrogens or androgens promoting tumour growth. The targeted modulation or blocking of these hormones has proven to be an effective form of therapy and is used in both adjuvant and palliative settings.

Anti-hormone therapy is an essential part of treatment for breast cancer , especially for hormone receptor-positive tumours. Tumours that express oestrogen and/or progesterone receptors can be inhibited in their growth by blocking the hormonal signalling pathways. The main approaches include the use of selective oestrogen receptor modulators (SERMs) such as tamoxifen , which blocks oestrogen receptors and thus inhibits the proliferative effect of oestrogens in breast tissue. Aromatase inhibitors such as anastrozole, letrozole or exemestane reduce oestrogen production in postmenopausal women by suppressing the conversion of androgens into oestrogens in peripheral tissue. These therapies are often used adjuvantly to reduce the risk of recurrence and can also be used in palliative therapy to control tumour growth in advanced stages.

Androgen deprivation therapy (ADT) is a key treatment approach for prostate cancer , as the growth of many prostate tumours is stimulated by testosterone and dihydrotestosterone (DHT). ADT is achieved through the surgical removal of the testicles (orchiectomy) or the medicinal suppression of testosterone production using gonadotropin-releasing hormone (GnRH) agonists or antagonists. GnRH agonists such as leuprorelin and goserelin lead to a permanent suppression of testosterone production after an initial hormone release. GnRH antagonists such as Degarelix block the receptor directly and avoid the initial hormone peak. In addition, androgen receptor antagonists such as enzalutamide or abiraterone, an inhibitor of androgen synthesis, can be used to further inhibit the effect of androgens on tumour cells.

Anti-hormone therapy is associated with specific side effects that are the result of hormonal suppression. Women treated with aromatase inhibitors or tamoxifen can often experience side effects such as hot flushes, vaginal dryness, muscle pain and an increased risk of osteoporosis . Tamoxifen is also associated with a slightly increased risk of venous thrombosis and endometrial cancer, especially with long-term use. Men on androgen deprivation therapy often experience side effects such as loss of libido, erectile dysfunction, loss of muscle mass, weight gain and an increased risk of osteoporosis and cardiovascular disease. These side effects can significantly impair quality of life and require careful monitoring and, if necessary, supportive measures such as the administration of bisphosphonates or denosumab to prevent bone loss.

Adjuvant hormone therapies are used to reduce the risk of recurrence after primary tumour treatment. In breast cancer , adjuvant anti-hormone therapy often lasts five to ten years, while in prostate cancer the duration of ADT varies depending on the risk profile. In the palliative setting, hormone therapy aims to slow tumour progression, alleviate symptoms and improve the patient's quality of life. For hormone-resistant tumours that no longer respond to standard therapy, innovative approaches such as combined hormone therapies, new inhibitors or immunotherapeutic strategies are being developed.

In summary, hormone therapy is an essential part of the treatment of hormone-dependent tumours. It is able to control tumour growth, improve quality of life and prevent relapses. Careful selection of therapy and monitoring of side effects are crucial to ensure the greatest possible benefit for patients, both in a curative and palliative context. The continued development of these therapies offers hope for improved treatment options for patients with hormone-dependent cancer.

Transgender medicine and hormone therapy

Gender reassignment hormone therapy is a central component of medical care for transgender people. It aims to harmonise the physical characteristics and hormonal profiles with the patient's gender identity and to improve their quality of life and psychological well-being. Hormone therapy can be used for both transgender women (male-to-female, MTF) and transgender men (female-to-male, FTM) and requires an individualised, evidence-based approach.

In transgender women, hormone therapy typically consists of the administration of oestrogens to induce feminising effects. These include the development of breast tissue, the redistribution of body fat into a feminine fat distribution pattern, the reduction of muscle mass and the softening of the skin. In addition, testosterone production is suppressed by the administration of antiandrogens such as spironolactone or cyproterone acetate. The focus is on lowering testosterone levels to the female reference range and adjusting oestrogen levels to the physiological values of cisgender women. In transgender men, testosterone is administered to promote masculinising changes. These include the development of facial and body hair, an increase in muscle mass, a deepening of the voice and a reduction in fatty tissue in the chest area. Testosterone levels are raised to the male reference range, with the therapy usually being carried out using intramuscular or transdermal preparations.

The long-term effects of gender reassignment hormone therapy are the subject of intensive research. Physical changes usually occur within the first two years, while the maximum effect often only becomes visible after several years. In the long term, hormone therapy leads to an improved quality of life, a reduction in gender dysphoria and positive effects on mental health, including a reduction in anxiety and depression. However, the potential risks and side effects must be carefully monitored. There is an increased risk of thromboembolic events with oestrogen therapies, particularly with the use of ethinylestradiol, which is generally avoided. Testosterone , on the other hand, can increase the risk of erythrocytosis and requires regular monitoring of the haematocrit. Regular monitoring of liver, heart and bone health is essential for both oestrogen and testosterone therapies.

Gender reassignment hormone therapy has profound psychological and social effects. It usually leads to a significant improvement in body satisfaction, strengthens self-confidence and facilitates social integration. Despite these positive effects, many transgender people continue to face challenges ranging from social stigmatisation to discrimination in medical and professional contexts. These aspects emphasise the need for comprehensive care that includes medical as well as psychological and social support.

Challenges and ethical issues play a central role in transgender medicine. One of the key challenges is to ensure equitable access to hormonal and surgical care. In many countries, there are still significant barriers, including financial barriers, a lack of qualified professionals and bureaucratic hurdles that make access to care difficult. Ethical issues also concern the autonomy and decision-making capacity of patients, particularly in the case of minors, where the initiation of puberty blockade or hormone therapy must be carefully considered. There is a tension between the protection of long-term health and the need to take early action to reduce gender dysphoria.

Paediatrics and puberty disorders

The treatment of growth disorders and delayed puberty in paediatrics requires a deep understanding of the endocrine mechanisms that control growth and pubertal development. Growth disorders can be caused by genetic, hormonal or systemic factors, while delayed puberty is usually due to inadequate activation of the hypothalamic-pituitary-gonadal axis. Targeted hormonal intervention plays a decisive role in both cases , especially in syndromes such as Turner and Klinefelter syndrome.

In the case of growth disorders, treatment is often aimed at promoting longitudinal growth and enabling the genetically predetermined final height to be reached. One of the main therapies is the administration of growth hormone (GH), particularly in children with documented growth hormone deficiency, Turner syndrome, chronic kidney disease or other growth disorders. Growth hormone works by promoting insulin -like-growth-factor-1 (IGF-1) production, which stimulates cell proliferation and bone growth plates. In Turner syndrome, which is characterised by a complete or partial loss of an X chromosome, growth hormone is often used in combination with oestrogens to promote growth and support pubertal development.

The treatment of delayed puberty requires careful consideration of the cause and the psychosocial effects of the delay. In adolescents with constitutional developmental delay, a common cause, hormonal intervention is not always necessary as puberty usually occurs spontaneously. However, if psychosocial stress is significant, short-term treatment with low doses of testosterone in boys or oestrogens in girls can help to induce puberty and reduce psychological stress. In the case of pathological causes such as hypogonadotropic hypogonadism , gonadotropic hormones or gonadotropin-releasing hormone (GnRH) therapies are used to stimulate endogenous hormone production and enable normal pubertal development.

Specific syndromes such as Turner and Klinefelter syndrome require customised treatment approaches. In Turner syndrome, oestrogens are used alongside growth hormone to induce and maintain puberty in order to promote the development of secondary sexual characteristics and bone density. In Klinefelter syndrome, which is characterised by the presence of an extra X chromosome in male patients, there is often a testosterone deficiency. Testosterone therapies are used to promote muscle mass, bone density and sexual development. In both syndromes, lifelong monitoring is necessary to avoid long-term complications such as cardiovascular disease or osteoporosis .

Early hormonal interventions can offer significant benefits but can also have long-term consequences. With growth hormone therapies, there is concern about potential effects on glucose homeostasis and an increased risk of certain cancers, although the evidence for this is limited. Hormonal induction of puberty may increase the risk of growth plate closure and reduced final height if inadequately monitored. Psychological consequences may also occur, particularly if expectations of treatment are not met or social and emotional problems persist due to the underlying condition.

Part III: Benefits, risks and controversies

Benefits of hormone therapy

Hormone therapy offers significant benefits in various medical contexts, as it specifically targets the regulation of hormonal imbalances. It makes a significant contribution to improving quality of life, preventing illness and providing support in specific phases of life in which hormonal changes play a central role.

The improvement in quality of life through hormone therapy is particularly noteworthy in conditions associated with a deficiency or dysregulation of hormones. For menopausal women , hormone replacement therapy (HRT) alleviates symptoms such as hot flushes, sleep disturbances, vaginal dryness and mood swings. These symptoms can significantly impair everyday function and well-being. The targeted supply of oestrogens, often in combination with progestins , restores hormonal balance, leading to a noticeable improvement in physical and psychological quality of life. In men with hypogonadism , testosterone replacement therapy restores libido, improves muscle mass and increases energy levels, which contributes to an improvement in quality of life and general well-being.

Disease prevention is another key benefit of hormone therapy. For example, hormone replacement therapy in postmenopausal women reduces the risk of osteoporosis and associated fractures, as oestrogens inhibit bone resorption and increase bone density. In specific groups, such as women with premature ovarian failure, hormone replacement therapy protects against the long-term consequences of oestrogen deficiency, including cardiovascular disease and cognitive impairment. By normalising testosterone levels in men, hormone therapy can also help to prevent metabolic diseases such as insulin resistance and lipid metabolism disorders, which are often associated with a testosterone deficiency. In paediatrics, targeted hormone therapy helps to correct growth disorders or pubertal developmental delays, which improves physical and mental health in the long term.

Hormone therapy also plays an important role in specific phases of life in which hormonal changes occur. During the reproductive phase, hormones can help to regulate cycle disorders or promote fertility, for example through ovulation induction in women with polycystic ovary syndrome (PCOS) or through gonadotropin therapy in men with hormone-induced infertility . In adolescence, hormone therapy is used to treat developmental disorders, for example delayed puberty or syndromes such as Turner and Klinefelter syndrome. In transgender medicine, gender reassignment hormone therapy is essential in order to adapt the physical characteristics to the gender identity, which not only achieves physical changes but also promotes psychological well-being and social integration.

Hormone therapy offers a wide range of benefits, from the treatment of acute symptoms to the prevention of long-term health complications. It improves quality of life, protects against serious illnesses and provides support during crucial phases of life in which hormonal changes play a central role. However, its effectiveness depends on individual adaptation, careful monitoring and continuous re-evaluation in order to optimally adapt the therapy to the patient's needs and minimise potential risks.

Risks and side effects

Hormone therapy, although of considerable benefit in many cases, is associated with specific risks and side effects that must be carefully considered. The most important risks include the risk of thrombosis, a potentially increased risk of certain types of cancer and other possible complications, which vary depending on the patient group and form of therapy.

A key risk of hormone therapy is the increased likelihood of thromboembolic events. This particularly affects women who receive systemic hormone replacement therapy (hormone replacement therapy) with oestrogens. The mechanism behind this risk lies in the procoagulant effect of oestrogens, which can increase the blood's tendency to clot. Studies show that the risk of venous thrombosis, such as deep vein thrombosis or pulmonary embolism, is higher with orally administered oestrogen preparations than with transdermal applications. Men receiving testosterone replacement therapy may also have an increased risk of thrombosis, especially if the therapy leads to erythrocytosis, which increases blood volume and viscosity.

Another significant risk relates to the development of hormone-dependent tumours. In women who receive combined hormone replacement therapy with oestrogens and progestogens , the risk of breast cancer is slightly increased, especially with long-term use beyond five years. Pure oestrogen therapies, which are often used in women without a uterus, appear to increase this risk less. With regard to endometrial cancer, there is an increased risk with insufficient progesterone supplementation, as oestrogens promote endometrial proliferation. For men receiving testosterone replacement therapy, concern about prostate cancer has long been a controversial issue. Recent studies suggest that well monitored therapy does not significantly increase the risk, but critical monitoring remains necessary.

In addition to these main complications, other side effects can also occur , such as cardiovascular risks, particularly in older patients or those with pre-existing risk factors. Long-term hormone therapies can have metabolic effects, such as influencing lipid metabolism, insulin sensitivity and liver function. Side effects such as sleep apnoea, acne or hair loss can occur with testosterone therapy , while water retention and breast tenderness are common with oestrogen therapies.

Weighing up the benefits and risks is essential and requires individual consideration of the patient. In younger postmenopausal women without significant risk factors, the benefits of hormone replacement therapy, particularly in terms of symptom relief and the prevention of osteoporosis, may outweigh the risks. However, for older women or those at increased risk of thrombosis, breast cancer or cardiovascular disease, caution is advised and alternative treatment strategies should be considered. In men with hypogonadism, the benefits of testosterone therapy often outweigh the risks, especially with careful monitoring of haematocrit and prostate health. Transgender individuals benefit significantly from gender reassignment hormone therapy, although monitoring of long-term side effects is essential to minimise potential risks such as cardiovascular complications.

With regard to the long-term effects of hormone therapy, we now know that these depend heavily on the patient group, the type of therapy and the duration of use. While many complications are well documented, research into long-term risks and potential late effects remains a dynamic field. The so-called "timing hypothesis" in hormone replacement therapy suggests that starting therapy at a younger age (within ten years of menopause) is associated with lower cardiovascular risks and better risk-benefit ratios than starting later. Long-term studies of testosterone therapy in men have shown that serious risks are rare when used and monitored appropriately, but the long-term effects on cardiovascular health and prostate cancer prevention require further investigation.

To summarise, hormone therapy has both significant benefits and specific risks that require individual and careful consideration. Modern evidence-based approaches, regular monitoring and consideration of patient-specific factors are essential to make therapy safe and effective. Long-term research remains necessary to deepen understanding of potential late effects and to further optimise treatment standards.

Controversies and social debates

The role of pharmaceutical companies in the popularisation of hormone therapy, particularly in the treatment of ageing processes, is complex and has both scientific and ethical implications. Pharmaceutical companies have contributed significantly to the further development and commercialisation of hormone replacement therapies, but not without controversy. In particular, the use of hormones in the anti-ageing market raises questions about misuse, scientific basis and ethical responsibility.

Pharmaceutical companies have improved the availability and effectiveness of hormone therapies through extensive research and development. In areas such as menopause and andropause treatment, they have developed products that have been proven to improve quality of life and prevent diseases such as osteoporosis or cardiovascular disease. At the same time, however, intensive marketing strategies have helped to present hormone therapy not only as a medical necessity, but also as a lifestyle treatment. Particularly in the 1990s, hormone replacement therapies for women were promoted as a "panacea" for a youthful appearance, energy and health, often without a differentiated presentation of potential risks. This marketing contributed to the widespread use of hormones, even in women without medical indications.

In the anti-ageing market, the abuse of hormones, particularly testosterone , growth hormone and DHEA (dehydroepiandrosterone), has become a growing problem. These substances are often marketed as a means of improving vitality, muscle mass and cognitive performance, although their long-term health benefits and risks in this context are insufficiently scientifically proven. Particularly problematic is that many anti-ageing practices take place outside of regulated medical care. Patients are often prescribed high doses of hormones without clear indications or regular monitoring. This not only leads to potentially serious side effects such as cardiovascular complications, hormonal imbalances and increased cancer risk, but also to a loss of trust in the medical community.

Scientific and ethical challenges affect both clinical research and the commercialisation of hormones. Scientifically, the evidence for many anti-ageing applications of hormones remains limited or contradictory. Clinical trials that comprehensively investigate potential benefits and risks are often expensive and time-consuming, which means that many claims about the benefits of hormonal anti-ageing treatments are not sufficiently supported by high-quality research. Ethically problematic is that in some cases uncertainties or gaps in knowledge are deliberately ignored in order to promote demand for these products.

Another ethical problem is the targeting of vulnerable groups. Menopausal women and older people in general are often target groups for aggressive marketing strategies that suggest to them that the natural ageing process is a "deficit" that needs to be corrected. This can lead not only to overtreatment, but also to increased social pressure to remain youthful and productive.

Pharmaceutical companies also have a responsibility to publish the results of clinical trials transparently, including the potential risks of hormone replacement therapies. Cases in which negative study results have been suppressed or trivialised have significantly undermined confidence in the industry. At the same time, independent studies such as the Women's Health Initiative (WHI), which highlighted the risks of hormone replacement therapy, have helped to clarify the indications for the therapy and focus on more personalised and safer use.

In summary, it can be said that pharmaceutical companies play an ambivalent role in the popularisation of hormone therapy. On the one hand, they contribute to the development of life-changing treatments; on the other hand, they sometimes encourage the misuse of hormones, particularly in the anti-ageing market, through aggressive marketing strategies and insufficient transparency. The scientific and ethical challenges require tighter regulation, a greater emphasis on evidence-based medicine and a critical examination of the long-term consequences of the commercialisation of hormones. This is essential to ensure patient safety and confidence in hormonal therapies.

Part IV: The future of hormone therapies

New developments and technologies

Hormone therapy is increasingly benefiting from new developments and technologies in molecular biology, genetics , precision medicine and innovative dosage forms such as nanotechnology. These advances enable more individualised and effective therapies that not only improve efficacy but also minimise side effects .

Advances in molecular biology and genetics have significantly deepened the understanding of hormonal signalling pathways. Technologies such as gene sequencing and CRISPR-Cas9 have made it possible to identify genetic variations that influence sensitivity to hormones or modulate the efficacy of hormone therapy. For example, specific genetic polymorphisms have been identified that influence the response to oestrogen or testosterone therapies. These findings could make it possible to treat patients in a targeted manner based on their genetic profile. In cancer research, molecular markers have been discovered that guide the choice of anti-hormone therapy in hormone-dependent tumours such as breast or prostate cancer . These markers make it possible to individualise therapies and identify resistance at an early stage, which significantly improves treatment strategies.

Precision medicine has the potential to revolutionise hormone therapy by enabling individually tailored treatment approaches. By combining genetic, epigenetic and metabolic information, customised therapies can be developed that are optimally tailored to the needs and biological conditions of the patient. For example, in the treatment of hormone-dependent breast cancer , the expression of oestrogen and progesterone receptors as well as HER2 is now taken into account in order to select a targeted therapy. Similar approaches could also be extended to other applications of hormone therapy, for example in the treatment of endocrine disorders or age-related hormonal changes.

Innovations in dosage form technology have made the administration of hormones safer, more effective and more user-friendly. Nanotechnology is playing an increasingly important role in this. With the help of nanoparticles, hormones can be transported to specific tissues or cells in a targeted manner, thereby reducing systemic side effects . This technology is being investigated, for example, in the development of drugs that have a maximum effect at a minimum dosage and significantly increase bioavailability. Liposomal formulations and polymer-based microcapsules offer the possibility of controlled release of hormones over longer periods of time, improving patient compliance Transdermal patches, microneedle systems and intranasal applications are further examples of innovative dosage forms that complement or replace traditional oral or intramuscular administration.

The combination of these advances opens up new perspectives for hormone therapy. For example, patients with hormone-dependent tumours could receive precise therapies that are tailored to their molecular profiles, while at the same time innovative technologies for targeted drug delivery could be used. In the treatment of endocrine disorders such as hypogonadism or menopause , individually adapted dosages and dosage forms could minimise the side effects and improve the quality of life of those affected.

In the long term, advances in artificial intelligence (AI) and data analytics are likely to play a key role by processing large amounts of clinical and genetic data and identifying patterns that enable the development of new therapies and the optimisation of existing approaches.

Alternative approaches

Alternative approaches such as the use of herbal phytohormones and lifestyle interventions are becoming increasingly important in the treatment of hormonal disorders . These approaches offer options that are often perceived as gentler alternatives to traditional hormone therapy. While herbal phytohormones are used in complementary medicine in particular, lifestyle changes can provide fundamental support in regulating hormonal imbalances.

Plant phytohormones are plant compounds that have a similar structure and function to human hormones, in particular oestrogens . Isoflavones , which are found in soya beans, red clover and other plants, and lignans, which are found in linseed, are the best known representatives. These compounds bind to oestrogen receptors and can have both an oestrogen-like effect (agonistic) and inhibit the effect of the body's own oestrogen (antagonistic), depending on the concentration and receptor type. Phytoestrogens are often used as an alternative to traditional hormone replacement therapy in the treatment of menopausal symptoms such as hot flushes and sleep disorders. Studies show that they can bring about moderate improvements in these symptoms, but their effectiveness remains limited compared to synthetic hormones. However, they are considered safer as they are not associated with an increased risk of breast cancer or thrombosis, although further research is needed to clarify long-term effects.

In addition to phytohormones, other herbal preparations such as monk's pepper, black cohosh and evening primrose oil also play a role in complementary medicine. These are mainly used for premenstrual syndrome (PMS), menopausal symptoms or irregular cycles. Although many users report positive effects, the scientific evidence for their effectiveness is often limited and the exact mechanisms of action are not fully understood. Nevertheless, they are an option for patients who prefer a natural approach or for whom synthetic hormone therapies are contraindicated.

Lifestyle interventions also play a central role in the prevention and treatment of hormonal disorders. Physical activity has a positive effect on hormone balance by improving insulin sensitivity, regulating cortisol levels and influencing the production of sex hormones. Regular exercise can help to stabilise hormone levels and improve symptoms such as irregular cycles or obesity, particularly in the case of polycystic ovary syndrome (PCOS). An active lifestyle can also help to increase natural testosterone levels and maintain muscle mass in men with age-related testosterone deficiency.

Diet also plays an important role in the regulation of hormonal functions. A balanced diet rich in unsaturated fatty acids, wholemeal products, fruit and vegetables supports hormone production and regulation. In particular, foods with a low glycaemic index can help to improve insulin sensitivity, which is of central importance in hormonal disorders such as PCOS or metabolic syndrome. In addition, an adequate intake of micronutrients such as vitamin D , magnesium and zinc can support endocrine function.

Stress management is another important aspect, as chronic stress increases cortisol levels and can dysregulate the hypothalamus, pituitary and adrenal axis (HPA axis). This dysregulation can have a negative effect on the production of sex hormones and thyroid function. Relaxation techniques such as yoga, meditation and mindfulness training can help to reduce stress and restore hormonal balance.

Phytohormones and lifestyle interventions offer valuable alternatives or supplements to conventional hormone therapies. While phytohormones and complementary approaches often have fewer side effects , their effectiveness remains limited compared to synthetic hormones. Lifestyle interventions such as exercise, diet and stress management, on the other hand, can play a central role in the prevention and treatment of hormonal imbalances by helping the body to regulate its hormonal balance in a natural way. However, these approaches require a high level of commitment and continuity from patients, which is why individual adaptation and counselling by specialists is essential.

Research perspectives

Hormone therapy research is a dynamic and interdisciplinary field that encompasses numerous open questions, innovative clinical approaches and technological possibilities. Long-term studies, new clinical strategies and the integration of big data and artificial intelligence (AI) play a crucial role in further improving the understanding and application of hormonal treatments.

Unanswered questions in hormone therapy concern both the mechanisms and the long-term effects. Despite extensive studies, it remains unclear why some patients respond better to hormonal therapies than others. The individual variability could be due to genetic differences, epigenetic changes or environmental factors, which underlines the need for personalised approaches.

The optimal duration and dosage of hormonal treatments is also not fully understood. In the case of hormone replacement therapy (HRT) for menopausal women, there is uncertainty about the long-term impact on cardiovascular disease, dementia and certain types of cancer. The risk-benefit profile of androgen therapy for men with age-related testosterone deficiency has also not yet been conclusively clarified, particularly with regard to prostate cancer and cardiovascular events.

Long-term studies are essential to better assess the safety and efficacy of hormonal treatments. Large cohort-based studies such as the Women's Health Initiative (WHI) have provided valuable insights, but have also sparked controversy. Future studies should aim to examine specific patient groups in more detail in order to develop differentiated recommendations for different age groups, genders and risk profiles. Randomised controlled trials (RCTs) could, for example, evaluate new hormone preparations, innovative combinations or alternative dosage forms in order to better understand both acute and long-term effects. In addition, preclinical studies are needed to further investigate the molecular basis of hormonal signalling pathways and to identify potential new target molecules.

New clinical approaches could be driven by advances in precision medicine. The integration of genetic and epigenetic data enables the development of customised therapies *that are* better tailored to the individual needs of patients. *The study of molecular biomarkers could help to identify patients* who benefit particularly from specific hormone therapies or those who are at increased risk of side effects . This is particularly relevant in hormone-dependent tumours such as breast or prostate cancer , where resistance to anti-hormone therapies is a major problem. Here, new approaches such as combination therapies or targeted drugs could improve efficacy and overcome resistance.

The importance of big data and artificial intelligence (AI) in hormone therapy research is growing rapidly. Large amounts of data from electronic health records, genetic databases and clinical studies offer the possibility of recognising patterns that would not be visible using traditional methods. AI-supported algorithms can help decipher complex relationships between genetic variations, hormonal profiles and treatment outcomes. Machine learning could also develop predictive models that calculate the probability of treatment success or side effects for individual patients. These approaches could also help to identify new target molecules or develop optimal dosages and treatment strategies.

Another exciting field is the use of AI for the discovery of new hormonal compounds. Molecule docking algorithms can be used to virtually test millions of potential compounds to identify those that interact with specific hormone receptors. This approach significantly speeds up the development process of new drugs and reduces costs. At the same time, predictive analyses could help to identify potential side effects at an early stage and thus increase the safety of new therapies.

Closing words

Hormone therapy is an essential part of modern medicine and covers a broad spectrum of applications ranging from the treatment of hormonal disorders to the support of specific phases of life. Its effectiveness is particularly evident in the improvement of quality of life, the prevention of diseases such as osteoporosis and the treatment of hormone-dependent tumours. Despite these successes, hormone therapies are not without risks. Thrombosis risks, possible cancer risks and other complications require careful consideration of the benefits and risks. However, advances in molecular biology, precision medicine and technology have helped to make these therapies more personalised, safer and more effective.

The future of hormone therapy is promising. The integration of big data and artificial intelligence will further deepen our understanding of the complex interactions in the endocrine system and enable personalised treatment approaches. Advances in genetics and epigenetics open up new possibilities for tailoring therapies precisely to the individual needs of patients. Technologies such as nanomedicine could revolutionise the dosage forms and effectiveness of hormonal treatments, while innovative research is potentially opening up new areas of application. At the same time, alternative approaches such as herbal phytohormones and lifestyle interventions will continue to play an important role, especially for patients who prefer natural or non-invasive options.

An appeal to the readership is of central importance: informed decisions are the key to safe and effective hormone therapy. This requires both sound information for patients and close interdisciplinary co-operation between doctors, researchers, pharmaceutical companies and political decision-makers. The focus should always be on customising therapy to the biological, social and psychological needs of patients. At the same time, it is essential to continue to critically question how scientific, technological and ethical aspects can be combined in practice in order to fully exploit the potential of hormone therapy and minimise possible risks.

To summarise, hormone therapy remains a fascinating and dynamic field of medicine that can improve the quality of life and health of many people with constant progress. However, its success depends crucially on how we translate the latest scientific findings into clinical practice while taking into account the individual needs and preferences of patients. The further development of these therapies is not only a challenge, but also an opportunity to push the boundaries of modern medicine and set new standards for personalised medicine.

Index